Praise

"*The Professor and the Madman* . . . is the linguistic detective story of the decade. . . . Winchester does a superb job of historical research that should entice readers even more interested in deeds than words."

—William Safire, *New York Times Magazine*

"Elegant and scrupulous." —*New York Times Book Review*

"I found *The Professor and the Madman* both enthralling and moving, in its brilliant reconstruction of a most improbable event: the major contributions made to the great *Oxford English Dictionary* by a deeply delusional, incarcerated 'madman,' and the development of a true friendship between him and the editor of the *OED*. One sees here the redemptive potential of work and love in even the most deeply, 'hopelessly,' psychotic." —Oliver Sacks, M.D.

"Remarkably readable, this chronicle of lexicography roams from the great dictionary itself to hidden nooks in the human psyche that sometimes house the motives for murder, the sources for sanity, and the blueprint for creativity."

—*Kirkus Reviews* (starred)

"An extraordinary tale, and Simon Winchester could not have told it better. . . . [He] has written a splendid book."

—*The Economist*

"[Winchester] has the journalistic virtues, including a talent for following things up and delving into unexpected corners."
—*New York Review of Books*

"A fascinating tale of madness, the evolution of dictionaries, Victorian England, eccentric autodidacts, and the likeness of two men who appear to be opposites. [It] is a compelling slice of social and intellectual history as well. Out of a near-forgotten fragment of history, Simon Winchester has created an evocative chronicle of the healing powers of affection upon the turmoil of a troubled mind."
—*Boston Globe*

"Singular, astonishing, and well-told from start to finish."
—*A Common Reader*

The Professor and
the Madman

Also by Simon Winchester

The Professor and the Madman

A Tale of Murder, Insanity, and the Making of the Oxford English Dictionary

Simon Winchester

FIRST HARPER PERENNIAL EDITION PUBLISHED 1999.
FIRST HARPER PERENNIAL OLIVE EDITION PUBLISHED 2016.

Illustrations by Philip Hood

The Library of Congress has catalogued the hardcover edition as follows:

Winchester, Simon.
    The professor and the madman : a tale of murder, insanity, and the making of the *Oxford English Dictionary*/Simon Winchester.—1st ed.
        p.   cm.
    Includes biographical references.
    ISBN 0-06-017596-6
    1. Oxford English dictionary.   2. Murray, James Augustus Henry, Sir, 1837–1915—Friends and associates.   3. United States—History—Civil War, 1861–1865—Veterans—Biography.   4. Psychiatric hospital patients—Great Britain—Biography.   5. New English dictionary on historical principals.   6. Lexicographers—Great Britain—Biography.   7. English language—Lexicography.   8. English language—Etymology.   9. Minor, William Chester.   I. Title.
PE1617.094W56   1998
423—dc21   98–10204

ISBN 978-0-06-256461-0 (Olive Edition)

16 17 18 19 20   RRD   10 9 8 7 6 5 4 3 2 1

To the memory of G. M.

Contents

Preface

Mysterious (mistī<ə>·riəs), *a*. [f. L. *mystērium* Mystery[1] + ous. Cf. F. *mystérieux*.]

1. Full of or fraught with mystery; wrapt in mystery; hidden from human knowledge or understanding; impossible or difficult to explain, solve, or discover; of obscure origin, nature, or purpose.

Popular myth has it that one of the most remarkable conversations in modern literary history took place on a cool and misty late autumn afternoon in 1896, in the small village of Crowthorne in the county of Berkshire.

One of the parties to the colloquy was the formidable Dr. James Murray, the editor of the *Oxford English Dictionary*. On the day in question he had traveled fifty miles by train from Oxford to meet an enigmatic figure named Dr. W. C. Minor, who was among the most prolific of the thousands of volunteer contributors whose labors lay at the core of the dictionary's creation.

For very nearly twenty years beforehand these two men had corresponded regularly about the finer points of English lexicography, but they had never met. Dr. Minor seemed never willing or able to leave his home at Crowthorne, never willing to come to Oxford. He was unable to offer any kind of explanation, or to do more than offer his regrets.

Dr. Murray, who himself was rarely free from the burdens of his work at his dictionary headquarters, the famous Scriptorium in Oxford, had nonetheless long dearly wished to see and thank his mysterious and intriguing helper. And particularly so by the late 1890s, with the dictionary well on its way to being half completed: Official honors were being showered upon all its creators, and Murray wanted to make sure that all those involved—even men so apparently bashful as Dr. Minor—were recognized for the valuable work they had done. He decided he would pay a visit.

Once he had made up his mind to go, he telegraphed his intentions, adding that he would find it most convenient to take a train that arrived at Crowthorne Station—then actually known as Wellington College Station, since it served the famous boys' school situated in the village—just after two on a certain Wednesday in November. Dr. Minor sent a wire by return to say that he was indeed expected and would be made most welcome. On the journey from Oxford the weather was fine; the trains were on time; the auguries, in short, were good.

At the railway station a polished landau and a liveried coachman were waiting, and with James Murray aboard they clip-clopped back through the lanes of rural Berkshire. After twenty minutes or so the carriage turned up a long drive lined with tall poplars, drawing up eventually outside a huge and rather forbidding red-brick mansion. A solemn servant showed the lexicographer upstairs, and into a book-lined study, where behind an immense mahogany desk stood a man of undoubted importance. Dr. Murray bowed gravely, and launched into the brief speech of greeting that he had so long rehearsed:

"A very good afternoon to you, sir. I am Dr. James Murray of the London Philological Society, and Editor of the *Oxford English Dictionary*. It is indeed an honour and a pleasure to at long last make your acquaintance—for you must be, kind sir, my most assiduous helpmeet, Dr. W. C. Minor?"

There was a brief pause, a momentary air of mutual embarrassment. A clock ticked loudly. There were muffled footsteps in the hall. A distant clank of keys. And then the man behind the desk cleared his throat, and he spoke:

"I regret, kind sir, that I am not. It is not at all as you suppose. I am in fact the Governor of the Broadmoor Criminal Lunatic Asylum. Dr. Minor is most certainly here. But he is an inmate. He has been a patient here for more than twenty years. He is our longest-staying resident."

Although the official government files relating to this case are secret, and have been locked away for more than a century, I have recently been allowed to see them. What follows is the strange, tragic, yet spiritually uplifting story they reveal.

The Dead of Night in Lambeth Marsh

Murder (mṵ·ɹdəɹ, *sb*. Forms: a. I morþor, -ur, 3–4 morþre, 3–4, 6 murthre, 4 myrþer, 4–6 murthir, morther, 5 *Sc*. murthour, murthyr, 5–6 murthur, 6 mwrther, *Sc*. morthour, 4–9 (now *dial*. and *Hist*. or *arch*.) murther; β. 3–5 murdre, 4–5 moerdre, 4–6 mordre, 5 moordre, 6 murdur, mourdre, 6– murder. [OE. *morðor* neut. (with pl. of masc. form *morþras*) = Goth. *maurþr* neut.:-OTeut. **murþro*ᵐ:–pre-Teut. *mrtro-m, f. root **mer-: mor-: mr-* to die, whence L. *morī* to die, *mors* (*morti-*) death, Gr. μορτός, βροτός mortal, Skr. *mṛ* to die, *mará* masc., *mrti* fem., death, *márta* mortal, OSl. *mьrěti*, Lith. *mirti* to die, Welsh *marw*, Irish *marþ* dead.

The word has not been found in any Teut. lang. but Eng. and Gothic, but that it existed in continental WGer. is evident, as it is the source of OF. *murdre, murtre* (mod. F. *meurtre*) and of med. L. *mordrum, murdrum*, and OHG. had the de-

rivative *murdren* MURDER *v.* All the Teut. langs.
exc. Gothic possessed a synonymous word from the
same root with different suffix: OE. *morð* neut.,
masc. (MURTH[1]), OS. *morð* neut., OFris. *morth,
mord* neut., MDu. *mort, mord* neut. (Du. *moord*),
OHG. *mord* (MHG. *mort*, mod. G. *mord*), ON.
morð neut.:–OTeut. **murþo-*:–pre-Teut. **mrto-*.

The change of original *ð* into *d* (contrary to the
general tendency to change *d* into *ð* before syllabic
r) was prob. due to the influence of the AF. *murdre,
moerdre* and the Law Latin *murdrum*.]

1. The most heinous kind of criminal homicide;
also, an instance of this. In *English* (also *Sc.* and
U.S.) *Law*, defined as the unlawful killing of a
human being with malice aforethought; often
more explicitly *wilful murder*.

In OE. the word could be applied to any homicide that was strongly reprobated (it had also
the senses 'great wickedness', 'deadly injury',
'torment'). More strictly, however, it denoted
secret murder, which in Germanic antiquity
was alone regarded as (in the modern sense) a
crime, open homicide being considered a private
wrong calling for blood-revenge or compensa-
tion. Even under Edward I, Britton explains the
AF. *murdre* only as felonious homicide of which
both the perpetrator and the victim are unidenti-
fied. The 'malice aforethought' which enters into

the legal definition of murder, does not (as now interpreted) admit of any summary definition. A person may even be guilty of 'wilful murder' without intending the death of the victim, as when death results from an unlawful act which the doer knew to be likely to cause the death of some one, or from injuries inflicted to facilitate the commission of certain offences. It is essential to 'murder' that the perpetrator be of sound mind, and (in England, though not in Scotland) that death should ensue within a year and a day after the act presumed to have caused it. In British law no degrees of guilt are recognized in murder; in the U.S. the law distinguishes 'murder in the first degree' (where there are no mitigating circumstances) and 'murder in the second degree'.

In Victorian London, even in a place as louche and notoriously crime-ridden as Lambeth Marsh, the sound of gunshots was a rare event indeed. The marsh was a sinister place, a jumble of slums and sin that crouched, dark and ogrelike, on the bank of the Thames just across from Westminster; few respectable Londoners would ever admit to venturing there. It was a robustly violent part of town as well—the footpad lurked in Lambeth, there had once been an outbreak of garroting, and in every crowded alley were the roughest kinds of pickpocket. Fagin, Bill Sikes, and Oliver Twist would have all seemed quite at home in Victorian Lambeth: This was Dickensian London writ large.

But it was not a place for men with guns. The armed criminal was a phenomenon little known in the Lambeth of Prime Minister Gladstone's day, and even less known in the entire metropolitan vastness of London. Guns were costly, cumbersome, difficult to use, hard to conceal. Then, as still today, the use of a firearm in the commission of a crime was thought of as somehow a very un-British act—and as something to be written about and recorded as a rarity. "Happily," proclaimed a smug editorial in Lambeth's weekly newspaper, "we in this country have no experience of the crime of 'shooting down,' so common in the United States."

So when a brief fusillade of three revolver shots rang out shortly after two o'clock on the moonlit Saturday morning of February 17, 1872, the sound was unimagined, unprecedented, and shocking. The three cracks—perhaps there were four—were loud, very loud, and they echoed through the cold and smokily damp night air. They were heard—and, considering their rarity, just by chance instantly recognized—by a keen young police constable named Henry Tarrant, then attached to the Southwark Constabulary's L Division.

The clocks had only recently struck two, his notes said later; he was performing with routine languor the duties of the graveyard shift, walking slowly beneath the viaduct arches beside Waterloo Railway Station, rattling the locks of the shops and cursing the bone-numbing chill.

When he heard the shots, Tarrant blew his whistle to alert any colleagues who (he hoped) might be on patrol nearby, and he began to run. Within seconds he had raced through the warren of mean and slippery lanes that made up what in those days was still called a village, and had emerged into the wide riverside swath of Belvedere Road, from whence he was certain the sounds had come.

Another policeman, Henry Burton, who had heard the piercing whistle, as had a third, William Ward, rushed to the scene. According to Burton's notes, he dashed toward the echoing sound and came across his colleague Tarrant, who was by then holding a man, as if arresting him. "Quick!" cried Tarrant. "Go to the road—a man has been shot!" Burton and Ward raced toward Belvedere Road and within seconds found the unmoving body of a dying man. They fell to their knees, and onlookers noted they had cast off their helmets and gloves and were hunched over the victim.

There was blood gushing onto the pavement—blood staining a spot that would for many months afterward be described in London's more dramatically minded papers as the location of A HEINOUS CRIME, A TERRIBLE EVENT, AN ATROCIOUS OCCURRENCE, A VILE MURDER.

The Lambeth Tragedy, the papers eventually settled upon calling it—as if the simple existence of Lambeth itself were not something of a tragedy. Yet this was a most unusual event, even by the diminished standards of the marsh dwellers. For though the place where the killing occurred had over the years been witness to many strange events, the kind

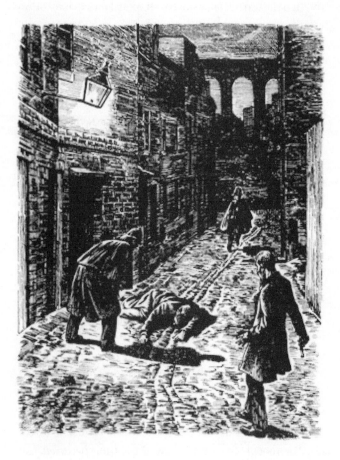

eagerly chronicled in the penny dreadfuls, this particular drama was to trigger a chain of consequences that was quite without precedent. And while some aspects of this crime and its aftermath would turn out to be sad and barely believable, not all of them, as this account will show, were to be wholly tragic. Far from it, indeed.

Even today Lambeth is a singularly unlovely part of the British capital, jammed anonymously between the great fan of roads and railway lines that take commuters in and out of the city center from the southern counties. These days the Royal Festival Hall and the South Bank Centre stand there, built on the site of the 1951 fairgrounds where an entertainment was staged to help cheer up the rationed and threadbare Londoners. Otherwise it is an unlovely, characterless sort of place—rows of prisonlike buildings that house lesser government ministries, the headquarters of an oil company around which winter winds whip bitterly, a few unmemorable pubs and newspaper shops, and the lowering presence of Waterloo Station—lately expanded with the terminal for the Channel Tunnel express trains—which exerts its dull magnetic pull over the neighborhood.

The railway chiefs of old never bothered to build a grand station hotel at Waterloo—though they did build monster structures of great luxury at the other London stations, like Victoria and Paddington, and even St. Pancras and King's Cross. Lambeth has long been one of the nastier parts of London; until very recently, with the further development of the Festival Hall site, no one of any style and consequence has ever wanted to linger there, neither a passenger back in the days of the Victorian boat trains, nor anyone for any reason at all today. It is slowly improving; but its reputation dogs it.

A hundred years ago it was positively vile. It was still then low, marshy, and undrained, a swampy gyre of pathways where a sad little stream called the Neckinger seeped into the Thames. The land was jointly owned by the archbishop of Canterbury and the duke of Cornwall, landlords who, rich enough in their own right, never bothered to develop it in the manner of the great lords of London—Grosvenor, Bedford, Devonshire—who created the squares, mansions, and terraces on the far side of the river.

So it was instead a place of warehouses, tenant shacks, and miserable rows of ill-built houses. There were blacking factories (shoe polish makers, like the one in which the young Charles Dickens worked) and soap boilers, small firms of dyers and lime burners, and tanning yards where the leatherworkers used a substance for darkening skins that was known as "pure" and that was gathered from the streets each night by the filthiest of the local indigents—"pure" being a Victorian term for dog turds.

A sickly smell of yeast and hops lay over the town, wafting from the chimneys of the great Red Lion Brewery, which stood on Belvedere Road, just north of the Hungerford Bridge. And this bridge was symbolic of what encompassed the entire marsh—the railways, hefted high over the swamps, on viaducts on which the trains (including those of the London Necropolis Railway, built to take corpses to the cemeteries in the suburb of Woking) chuffed and snorted, and across which miles of wagons lurched and banged. Lambeth was widely regarded as one of the noisiest and most sulfurous parts of a capital that had already a grim reputation for din and dirt.

Lambeth Marsh was also, as it happened, just beyond the legal jurisdiction of both the Cities of London and Westminster. It belonged administratively—at least until 1888—to the County of Surrey—meaning that the relatively strict laws that applied to the capital's citizens did not apply to anyone who ventured, via one of the new bridges, like Waterloo, Blackfriars, Westminster, or Hungerford, into the wen of Lambeth. The village thus fast became known as a site of revelry and abandon—a place where public houses, brothels, and lewd theaters abounded, and where a man could find entertainment of all kinds—and disease of all varieties—for no more than a handful of pennies.

To see a play that would not pass muster with the London censors, to be able to drink absinthe into the small hours of the morning, to buy the choicest pornography newly smuggled from Paris, or to have a girl of any age and not be concerned that a Bow Street runner (as London's early police were known), or her parents, might chase after you—you "went Surreyside," as they said, to Lambeth.

But, as with most slums, its cheapness attracted respectable men to live and work in Lambeth too, and by all accounts George Merrett was one of them. He was a stoker at the Red Lion Brewery; he had been there for the previous eight years, employed all the time as one of the gang who kept the fires burning through the day and night, keeping the vats bubbling and the barley malting. He was thirty-four years old and he lived locally, at 24 Cornwall Cottages, on the Cornwall Road.

George Merrett was, like so many younger workers in Victorian London, an immigrant from the countryside, and so was his wife, Eliza. He came from a village in Wiltshire, she from Gloucestershire. They had both been farm laborers and—with no protection by unions, no solidarity with their fellows—had been paid trifling sums to perform humiliating tasks for pitiless masters. They had met at a farm show in the Cotswolds and had vowed to leave together for the immeasurable possibilities offered by London, only two hours away on the new express train from Swindon. They moved first to north London, where their first daughter, Clare, was born in 1860; then they shifted into the city center; and finally in 1867, the family having become too large and costly and manual work too scarce, they found themselves near the brewery site in the bustling sty of Lambeth.

The young couple's surroundings and lodgings were exactly as the illustrator Gustave Doré had drawn on one of his horrified expeditions from Paris: a dim world of bricks and soot and screeching iron, of huddled tenements, of tiny backyards, each with a privy and clothes boiler and washing line, and everywhere an air of damp and sulfurous stench, and even a rough-hewn, rollicking, hugger-mugger, devil-may-care, peculiarly London type of good cheer. Whether the Merretts missed the fields and the cider and the skylarks, or whether they imagined that that ideal had ever truly been the world they had left, we shall never know.

By the winter of 1871 George and Eliza had, as was typical of the inhabitants of the dingier quarters of Victorian London, a very substantial family: six children, ranging from Clare at nearly thirteen to Freddy at twelve months. Mrs. Merrett was about to be confined with her seventh pregnancy. They were a poor family, as were most in Lambeth: George Merrett brought home twenty-four shillings a week, a miserable sum even then. With rent payable to the archbishop, and with food needed for the eight ever-open mouths, theirs were straitened circumstances indeed.

On the Saturday morning, just before 2 A.M., Merrett was awakened by a neighbor tapping on his window, as prearranged. He rose from bed, and readied himself for the dawn shift. It was a bitter morning, and he dressed as warmly as he could afford: a threadbare greatcoat over the kind of smock-jacket that Victorians called a slop, a tattered gray shirt, corduroy trousers tied at the ankle with twine, heavy socks, and black boots. The clothes were none too clean, but he was to heave coal for the next eight hours, and could not be too bothered with appearance.

His wife recalled him striking a light before leaving home. Her last sight of him was under one of the bright gas-lamps with which Lambeth's streets had recently been equipped. His breath was visible in the cold night air—or maybe he was just puffing on his pipe—and he walked purposefully down to the end of Cornwall Road before turning into Belvedere Road. The night was clear and starlit and, once his footsteps had faded, soundless except for the clanking and puffing of the ever-present railway engines.

Mrs. Merrett had no reason to be concerned: She assumed, as she had for each of the twenty previous nights on which her husband had worked the dawn shift, that all would be well. George was simply making his way as usual toward the high walls and ornate gates of the great brewery where he worked, shoveling coal beneath the shadow of the great red lion that was one of London's better-known landmarks. There may have been little money in the job; but working at so famous an institution as the Red Lion Brewery, well, that was some reason for pride.

But that night George Merrett never reached his destination. As he passed the entrance to Tennison Street, between where the south side of the Lambeth Lead Works abutted onto the north wall of the brewery, there came a sudden cry. A man shouted at him, appeared to be chasing him, was yelling furiously. Merrett was frightened: This was something more than a mere footpad—that silent and menacing figure who lurked in the dark carrying a lead-tipped cosh and wearing a mask; this was something quite out of the ordinary, and Merrett began to run in terror, slipping and sliding on the frost-slick cobbles. He looked back: The man was still there, still chasing after him, still shouting angrily. Then, quite incredibly, he stopped and raised a gun, took aim, and fired.

The shot missed, whistling past him and striking the brewery wall. George Merrett tried to run faster. He cried out for help. There was another shot. Perhaps another. And then a final shot that struck the unfortunate Merrett in the neck. He fell heavily onto the cobbled pavement, his face down, a pool of blood spreading around him.

Moments later came the running footfalls of Constable Burton, who found the man, lifted him, and attempted to comfort him. The other policeman, William Ward, summoned a passing hansom cab from the still-busy thoroughfare of Waterloo Road. They gently picked the wounded man up from the ground, hoisted him into the vehicle, and ordered the driver to take them as fast as possible to St. Thomas's Hospital, five hundred yards farther south on Belvedere Road, across from the archbishop's London palace. The horses did their best, their hooves striking sparks from the cobbles as they rushed the victim to the emergency entrance.

It was a futile journey. Doctors examined George Merrett and attempted to close the gaping wound in his neck. But his carotid artery had been severed, his spine snapped by two large-caliber bullets.

The man who had perpetrated this unprecedented crime was, within moments of committing it, in the firm custody of Constable Tarrant. He was a tall, well-dressed man of what the policeman described as "military appearance," with an erect bearing and a haughty air. He held a still-smoking revolver in his right hand. He made no attempt to run but stood silently as the policeman approached.

"Who is it that has fired?" asked the constable.

"I did," said the man, holding up the gun. Tarrant snatched it from him.

"Whom did you fire at?" he asked.

The man pointed down Belvedere Road, to the figure lying motionless beneath a street lamp just outside the brewery store. He made the only droll remark that history records him as having made—but a remark that, as it happens, betrayed one of the driving weaknesses of his life.

"It was a man," he said, with a tone of disdain. "You do not suppose I would be so cowardly as to shoot a *woman!*"

By now two other policemen had arrived on the scene, as had inquisitive locals—among them the Hungerford Bridge toll collector, who at first had not dared go out "for fear I would take a bullet," and a woman undressing in her room on Tennison Street—a street in which it was apparently far from uncommon for women to be undressing at all hours. Constable Tarrant, pointing toward the victim and ordering his two colleagues to see what they could do for him and to prevent a crowd from gathering, escorted the supposed—and unprotesting—murderer to the Tower Street police station.

On the way his prisoner became rather more voluble, though Tarrant described him as cool, collected, and clearly not affected by drink. It had all been a terrible accident; he had shot the wrong man, he insisted. He was after someone else, someone quite different. Someone had broken into his room; he was simply chasing him away, defending himself as anyone surely had a perfect right to do.

"Don't handle me!" he said, when Tarrant put a hand on his shoulder. But then, rather more gently, he said to the policeman: "You have not searched me, you know."

"I'll do that at the station," replied the constable.

"How do you know I haven't got another gun, and might shoot you?"

The policeman, plodding and imperturbable, replied

that if he did have another gun, perhaps he would be so kind as to keep it in his pocket for the time being.

"But I do have a knife," replied the prisoner.

"Keep that in your pocket also," said the stolid constable.

There turned out to be no other gun, but a search did turn up a long hunting knife in a leather sheath, strapped to the man's belt behind his back.

"A surgical instrument," it was explained. "I don't always carry it with me."

Tarrant, once he had completed the search, explained to the desk sergeant what had happened on Belvedere Road a few moments before. The pair then set about formally interviewing the arrested man.

His name was William Chester Minor. He was thirty-seven years old, and, as the policemen suspected from his bearing, a former army officer. He was also a qualified surgeon. He had lived in London for less than a year and had taken rooms locally, living alone in a simple furnished upstairs room nearby at 41 Tennison Street. He evidently had no financial need to live so economically, for he was in fact a man of very considerable means. He hinted that he had come to this lubricious quarter of town for reasons other than the simply monetary, though what those reasons might be did not emerge in the early interrogations. By dawn he was taken off to the Horsemonger Lane jail, charged with murder.

But there was one additional complication. William Minor, it turned out, came from New Haven, Connecticut. He had a commission in the U.S. Army. He was an American.

This put a wholly new complexion on the case. The American legation had now to be told: And so in midmorning, despite its being a Saturday, the Foreign Office formally notified the U.S. Minister in London that one of their army surgeons had been arrested and was being held on a charge of murder. The shooting on Belvedere Road, Lambeth—already because of its rarity a cause célèbre—had now become an international incident.

The British papers, always eager to vent editorial spleen on their transatlantic rivals, made hay with this particular aspect of the story.

"The light estimation in which human life is held by Americans," sniffed the *South London Press*,

> may be noted as one of the most significant points of difference between them and Englishmen, and this is a most shocking example of it brought to our own doors. The victim of a cruel mistake has left a wife near confinement, and seven children, the eldest only thirteen, to the mercy of the world. It is gratifying to be able to record that the benevolent are coming forward with alacrity to the succour of the widow and the fatherless, and it is most sincerely to be hoped that all who can spare even a trifle will do their best to help the victims of this dreadful tragedy. The American Vice-Consul General has, in the most thoughtful manner, opened a subscription list, and issued an appeal to Americans now in London to do

what they can to alleviate the misery which an act of their countryman's has entailed.

Scotland Yard detectives were soon put onto the case, so important had it suddenly become that justice was seen to be done on both sides of the Atlantic. Since Minor, silent in his prison cell, was offering no help except to say that he did not know the victim and had shot him in error, they began to investigate any possible motive. In doing so they uncovered the beginnings of the trail of a remarkable and tragic life.

William Minor had come to Britain the previous autumn, because he was ill—suffering at least in part from an ailment some papers said "was occasioned by the looseness of his private life." It was suggested by the lawyer later appointed to defend him that his motivation in coming to England was to quiet a mind that had become, as Victorian doctors were apt to say, "inflamed." It was said that he had suffered "a lesion on the brain," and many causes were put forward for it. He had, according to his lawyer, been in an asylum in the United States, and he had taken retirement from the army on the grounds of ill health. He had been described by those who met him as "a gentleman of fine education and ability, but with eccentric and dissolute habits."

He first settled at Radley's Hotel, in the West End, and from there traveled by train to the major cities of Europe. He had brought with him a letter from a friend at Yale University, recommending him to John Ruskin, the celebrated Brit-

ish artist and critic. The two men had met once, and Minor
had been encouraged to take his watercolors along with him
on his travels, and to paint as a form of relaxation.

As the police imagined, Minor had moved from the West
End shortly after Christmas 1871, and settled in Lambeth—a
highly dubious choice for a man of his background and
breeding unless, as he later admitted, it offered him easy access to easy women. The American authorities told Scotland
Yard that they already had records of his behavior as an army
officer: He had a long history of frequenting what were then
beginning to be called the "Tenderloin Districts" of the cities
in which he had been posted—most notably New York, where
he had been assigned to Governor's Island and from where,
on his leave days, he had gone regularly to some of Manhattan's roughest bars and music halls. He had, it was said, a
prodigious sexual appetite. He had caught venereal diseases
at least once, and a medical examination conducted at Horsemonger Lane jail showed that he had a case of gonorrhea even
then. He had caught it, he said, from a local prostitute, and
had tried to cure it by injecting white Rhine wine into his
urethra—an almost amusingly inventive attempt at a remedy, and one that, not surprisingly, failed.

His room, however, betrayed none of this seamier side.
The detectives reported that they found his heavy leather-
and-brass-bound portmanteaus, a great deal of money—
mainly French, in twenty-*livre* notes—a gold watch and
chain, some Eley's bullets for his gun, his surgeon's commission, and his letter of appointment as a captain in the U.S.
Army. There was also the letter of introduction to Ruskin,

as well as a large number of watercolors, evidently by Minor himself. They were said by everyone who saw them to be of the highest quality—views of London, largely, many from the hills above the Crystal Palace.

His landlady, Mrs. Fisher, said that he had been a perfectly good tenant, but odd. He used to go away for several days at a time, and on returning, rather ostentatiously left his hotel bills—the Charing Cross Hotel was one she remembered, the Crystal Palace Hotel another—lying around for all to see. He seemed, she said, a very anxious man. Often he demanded that the furniture in his room be moved. He also seemed afraid that people might break in.

He had one particular worry, Mrs. Fisher told the police: Doctor Minor was apparently formidably afraid of the Irish. He would ask interminably whether or not she had any Irish servants working in the house—and if so, demand that they be sacked. Did she have Irish visitors, any Irish lodgers? He was always to be kept informed—of a possibility that in Lambeth (which had a large population of casual Irish laborers, working on the legions of London construction sites) was in fact all too real.

Yet it was not until the murder trial, held in early April, that the full extent of Doctor Minor's illness became starkly apparent. Among the score of witnesses who appeared before the lord chief justice in the court at Kingston Assizes—for this was Surrey's jurisdiction still, not London's—three of them told a stunned courtroom what they knew of the sad captain.

The London police, for a start, admitted that they were already somewhat acquainted with him, and that for some time before the murder had known that they had a troubled man living in their midst. A Scotland Yard detective named Williamson testified that Minor had come to the Yard three months earlier, complaining that men were coming to his rooms at night, trying to poison him. He thought that they were members of the Fenian Brotherhood—militant Irish nationalists—and they were bent on breaking into his lodgings, hiding in the roof rafters, slipping through the windows.

He made such allegations several times, said Williamson; shortly before Christmas, Minor had even persuaded the commissioner of police in New Haven to write a letter to the Yard, underlining the fears that Minor felt. Even after the doctor moved to Tennison Street, he kept in touch with Williamson—on January 12, 1872, he wrote that he had been drugged and was afraid that the Fenians were planning to murder him and make it look as though his death had been a suicide.

A classic cry for help, one might think today. But an exasperated Superintendent Williamson did nothing and told no one, beyond noting with some contempt in his logbook that Minor was clearly—and this was the first use of the word to describe the hapless American—insane.

Then came a witness who had something very curious to offer from his observations of Doctor Minor during the time the American was held on remand in the cells at Horsemonger Lane.

The witness, whose name was William Dennis, was a

member of a profession that has long since receded from modern memory: He was what was called a "Bethlem watcher." Usually he was employed at London's Bethlehem Hospital for the Insane—such a dreadful place that the name has given us the word *bedlam*—where his duties included watching the prisoner-patients through the night to make sure that they behaved themselves and did not try to cheat justice by committing suicide. He had been seconded to the Horsemonger Lane Jail in mid-February, he said, to watch the nocturnal activities of the strange visitor. He had watched him, he testified, for twenty-four nights.

It was a most curious and disturbing experience, Dennis told the jury. Each morning Doctor Minor would awake and immediately accuse him of having been paid by someone specifically to molest him while he slept. Then he would spit, dozens of times, as though trying to remove something that had been put into his mouth. He would next leap from his bed and scrabble about underneath it, looking for people who, he insisted, had hidden there and were planning to annoy him. Dennis told his superior, the prison surgeon, that he was quite certain William Minor was mad.

From the police interrogation notes came the evidence of an imagined motive for the crime—and with them a further indication of Doctor Minor's patent instability. Each night, Minor had told his questioners, unknown men—often lower-class, often Irish—would come to his room while he was sleeping. They would maltreat him; they would violate him in ways he could not possibly describe. For months, ever since these nocturnal visitors had begun to torment him, he had taken to sleeping with his Colt service revolver, loaded with five cartridges, beneath his pillow.

On the night in question he awoke with a start, certain that a man was standing in the shadows at the foot of his bed. He reached under the pillow for his gun; the man saw him and took to his heels, running down the stairs and out of the house. Minor followed him as fast as he could, saw a man running down into Belvedere Road, was certain that this was the intruder, shouted at him, then fired four times, until he had hit him and the man lay still, unable to harm him further.

The court listened in silence. The landlady shook her head. No one could get into her house at night without a key, she had said. Everyone slept very lightly; there could not have been an intruder.

And as final confirmation the court then heard from the prisoner's stepbrother, George Minor. It had been a nightmare, said George, having brother William staying in the family house in New Haven. Every morning he would accuse people of trying to break into his room the night before, trying to molest him. He was being persecuted. Evil men were trying to insert metallic biscuits, coated with poison, in his mouth. They were in league with others who hid in the attic, came down at night while he was asleep, and treated him foully. Everything was punishment, he said, for an act he had been forced to commit while in the American army. Only by going to Europe, he said, could he escape his demons. He would travel and paint and live the life of a respected gentleman of art and culture—and the persecutors might melt away into the night.

The court listened in melancholy silence while Doctor Minor sat in the dock, morose, shamed. The lawyer the American consul-general had procured for him said only that it was clear that his client was insane, and that the jury should treat him as such.

The chief justice nodded his agreement. It had been a brief but sorry case, the defendant an educated and cultured man, a foreigner and a patriot, a figure quite unlike the wretches who more customarily stood in the dock before him. But the law had to be applied with just precision, whatever the condition or estate of the defendant; and the decision in this affair was in a sense a foregone conclusion.

For thirty years the law in such cases had been guided by what were known as the McNaughton rules—named for the man who, in 1843, shot dead Sir Robert Peel's secretary, and who was acquitted on the grounds that he was so mad he could not tell right from wrong. The rules, which judged criminal responsibility rather than guilt, were to be applied in this case, he told the jury. If they were convinced that the prisoner was "of unsound mind" and had killed George Merrett while under some delusion of the kind that they had just heard about, then they must do as juries were wont to do in this extraordinarily lenient time in British justice: They were to find William Chester Minor not guilty, on grounds of insanity, and leave the judge to apply such custodial sanction as he felt prudent and necessary.

And that is what the jury did, without deliberation, late on the afternoon of April 6, 1872. They found Doctor Minor legally innocent of a murder that all—including him—knew that he had committed. The lord chief justice then applied the only sentence that was available to him—a sentence still passed occasionally today, and that has a beguiling charm to its language, despite the swingeing awfulness of its connotations.

"You will be detained in safe custody, Dr. Minor," said the judge, "until Her Majesty's Pleasure be known." It was a decision that was to have unimaginable and wholly unanticipated implications, effects that echo and ripple through the English literary world to this day.

The Home Department took brief note of the sentence and made the further decision that Doctor Minor's detention—which, considering the severity of his illness, was likely to occupy the rest of his natural life—would have to be suffered in the newly built showpiece of the British penal system, a sprawling set of red-brick buildings located behind high walls and spiked fences in the village of Crowthorne, in the Royal County of Berkshire. Doctor Minor was to be transported as soon as was convenient from his temporary prison in Surrey to the Asylum for the Criminally Insane, Broadmoor.

Dr. William C. Minor, surgeon-captain, U.S. Army, a forlornly proud figure from one of the oldest and best-regarded families of New England, was henceforward to be formally designated in Britain by Broadmoor File Number 742, and to be held in permanent custody as a "certified criminal lunatic."

2

The Man Who Taught Latin to Cattle

Polymath (pɒ·limæþ′), *sb. (a.)* Also 7 **polumathe.** [ad. Gr. πολυμαθής having learnt much, f. πολυ- much + μαθ-, stem of μανθάνειν to learn. So F. *polymathe.*] A person of much or varied learning; one acquainted with various subjects of study.

1621 BURTON *Anat. Mel.* Democr. to Rdr. (1676) 4/2 To be thought and held Polumathes and Polyhistors. *a* **1840** MOORE *Devil among Schol.* 7 The Polymaths and Polyhistors, Polyglots and all their sisters. **1855** M. PATTISON *Ess.* I. 290 He belongs to the class which German writers . . . have denominated 'Polymaths'. **1897** O. Smeaton *Smollett* ii. 30 One of the last of the mighty Scots polymaths.

Philology (filɒ·lŏdʒi). [In Chaucer, ad. L. *philologia*; in 17th c. prob. a. F. *philologie*, ad. L. *philologia*, a. Gr. Φιλολογία, abstr. sb. from Φιλόλογος fond of speech, talkative; fond of discussion or argument; studious of words; fond of learning and literature, literary; f. *Φιλο-* PHILO- + *λόγος* word, speech, etc.]

1. Love of learning and literature; the study of literature, in a wide sense, including grammar, literary criticism and interpretation, the relation of literature and written records to history, etc.; literary or classical scholarship; polite learning.

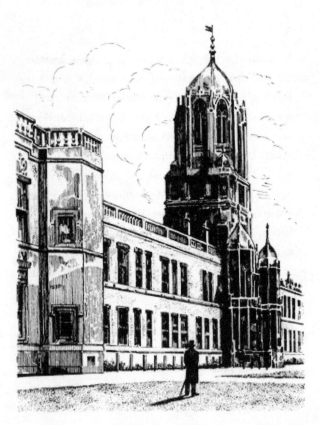

It took more than seventy years to create the twelve tomb-stone-size volumes that made up the first edition of what was to become the great *Oxford English Dictionary*. This heroic, royally dedicated literary masterpiece—which was first called the *New English Dictionary*, but eventually became the *Oxford* ditto, and thenceforward was known familiarly by its initials as the *OED*—was completed in 1928; over the following years there were five supplements and then, half a century later, a second edition that integrated the first and all the subsequent supplementary volumes into one new twenty-volume whole. The book remains in all senses a truly monu-mental work—and with very little serious argument is still regarded as a paragon, the most definitive of all guides to the language that, for good or ill, has become the lingua franca of the civilized modern world.

Just as English is a very large and complex language, so the *OED* is a very large and complex book. It defines well over half a million words. It contains scores of millions of charac-ters, and, at least in its early versions, many miles of hand-set type. Its enormous—and enormously heavy—volumes are bound in dark blue cloth: Printers and designers and bookbinders worldwide see it as an apotheosis of their art, a handsome and elegant creation that looks and feels more than amply suited to its lexical thoroughness and accuracy.

The *OED*'s guiding principle, the one that has set it apart from most other dictionaries, is its rigorous dependence on gathering quotations from published or otherwise recorded

uses of English and using them to illustrate the use of the
sense of every single word in the language. The reason behind this unusual and tremendously labor-intensive style of
editing and compiling was both bold and simple: By gathering and publishing selected quotations, the dictionary
could demonstrate the full range of characteristics of each
and every word with a very great degree of precision. Quotations could show exactly how a word has been employed
over the centuries; how it has undergone subtle changes of
shades of meaning, or spelling, or pronunciation; and, perhaps most important of all, how and more exactly *when* each
word slipped into the language in the first place. No other
means of dictionary compilation could do such a thing: Only
by finding and showing examples could the full range of a
word's past possibilities be explored.

The aims of those who began the project, back in the
1850s, were bold and laudable, but there were distinct commercial disadvantages to their methods: It took an immense
amount of time to construct a dictionary on this basis, it was
too time-consuming to keep up with the evolution of the
language it sought to catalog, the work that finally resulted
was uncommonly vast and needed to be kept updated with
almost equally vast additions, and it remains to this day for
all of these reasons a hugely expensive book both to produce
and to buy.

But withal it is widely accepted that the *OED* has a value
far beyond its price; it remains in print, and it still sells well.
It is the unrivaled cornerstone of any good library, an essential work for any reference collection. And it is still cited

as a matter of course—"the *OED* says"—in parliaments, courtrooms, schools, and lecture halls in every corner of the English-speaking world, and probably in countless others beyond.

It wears its status with a magisterial self-assurance, not least by giving its half million definitions a robustly Victorian certitude of tone. Some call the language of the dictionary old-fashioned, high-flown, even arrogant. Note well, they say by way of example, how infuriatingly prissy the compilers remain when dealing with even so modest an oath as "bloody": Though the modern editors place the original *NED* definition between quotation marks—it is a word "now constantly in the mouths of the lowest classes, but by respectable people considered 'a horrid word', on a par with obscene or profane language, and usually printed in the newspapers (in police reports, etc.) 'b——y'"—even the modern definition is too lamely self-regarding for most: "There is no ground for the notion," the entry reassures us, "that 'bloody', offensive as from associations it now is to ears polite, contains any profane allusion. . . ."

It is those with "ears polite," one supposes, who see in the dictionary something quite different: They worship it as a last bastion of cultured Englishness, a final echo of value from the greatest of all modern empires.

But even they will admit of a number of amusing eccentricities about the book, both in its selections and in the editors' choice of spellings; a small but veritable academic industry has recently developed in which modern scholars grumble about what they see as the sexism and racism of the work, its fussily and outdated imperial attitude. (And to Oxford's undying shame there is even one word—though only one—that all admit was actually *lost* during the seven decades of the *OED*'s preparation—though the word was added in a supplement, five years after the first edition appeared.)

There are many such critics, and with the book being such a large and immobile target there will no doubt be many more. And yet most of those who come to use it, no matter how doctrinally critical they may be of its shortcomings, seem duly and inevitably, in the end, to admire it as a work of literature, as well as to marvel at its lexicographical scholarship. It is a book that inspires real and lasting affection: It is an awe-inspiring work, the most important reference book ever made, and, given the unending importance of the English language, probably the most important that is ever likely to be.

The story that follows can fairly be said to have *two* protagonists. One of them is Doctor Minor, the murdering soldier from the United States, and there is one other. To say that a story has two protagonists, or three, or ten, is a perfectly acceptable, unremarkable modern form of speech. It happens, however, that a furious lexicographical controversy once raged over the use of the word—a dispute that helps illustrate the singular and peculiar way in which the *Oxford English Dictionary* has been constructed and how, when it flexes its muscles, it has a witheringly intimidating authority.

The word *protagonist* itself—when used in its general sense of meaning the leading figure in the plot of a story, or in a competition, or as the champion of some cause—is common enough. It is, as might be expected of a familiar word, defined fully and properly in the dictionary's first edition of 1928.

The entry begins with the customary headings that show its spelling, its pronunciation, and its etymology (it comes from the Greek [πρῶτος] meaning "first" and [ἀγωνιστής] meaning "actor" or, literally, the leading character to appear in a drama). Following this comes the distinguishing additional feature of the *OED*—the editors' selection of a string of six supporting quotations—which is about the average number for any one *OED* word, though some merit many more. The editors have divided the quotations under two headings.

The first heading, with three sources quoted, shows how the word has been used to mean, literally, "the chief personage in a drama"; the next three quotations demonstrate a subtle difference, in which the word means "the leading personage in any contest," or "a prominent supporter . . . of any cause." By general consent this second meaning is the more modern; the first is the older and now somewhat archaic version.

The oldest quotation used to illustrate the first of these two meanings was that tracked down by the dictionary's lexical detectives from the writings of John Dryden in 1671. "'Tis charg'd upon me," the quotation reads, "that I make debauch'd Persons . . . my protagonists, or the chief persons of the drama."

This, from a lexicographical point of view, seems to be the English word's mother lode, a fair clue that the word may well have been introduced into the written language in that year, and possibly not before. (But the *OED* offers no guar-

antee. German scholars in particular are constantly deriv-
ing much pleasure from winning an informal lexicographic
contest that aims at finding quotations that antedate those
in the *OED*: At last count the Germans alone had found
thirty-five thousand instances in which the *OED* quotation
was *not* the first; others, less stridently, chalk up their own
small triumphs of lexical sleuthing, all of which Oxford's editors accept with disdainful equanimity, professing neither
infallibility nor monopoly.)

This single quotation for *protagonist* is peculiarly neat,
moreover, in that Dryden explicitly states the newly minted
word's meaning within the sentence. So from the dictionary
editors' point of view there is a double benefit, of having the
word's origin dated and its meaning explained, and both by
a single English author.

Finding and publishing quotations of usage is an imper-
fect way of making pronouncements about origins and meanings, of course—but to nineteenth-century lexicographers it
was the best method that had yet been devised—and it has
not yet been bettered. From time to time experts succeed
in challenging specific findings like this, and on occasions
the dictionary is forced to recant, is obliged to accept a new
and earlier quotation and give to a particular word a longer
history than the Oxford editors first allowed. Happily *protagonist* itself has not so far been successfully challenged on
chronological grounds. So far as the *OED* is concerned, 1671
still stands: The word has for three hundred odd years been
a member of that giant corpus known as the English vocabulary.

The word appears again, and with a new supporting quotation, in the 1933 *Supplement*—a volume that had to be added because of the sheer weight of new words and new evidence of new meanings that had accumulated during the decades when the original dictionary was being compiled. By now another shade of meaning had been found for it—that of "a leading player in some game or sport." A sentence supporting this, from a 1908 issue of *The Complete Lawn Tennis Player*, is produced in evidence.

But then comes the controversy. The other great book on the English language, Henry Fowler's hugely popular *Modern English Usage*, which was first published in 1926, insisted—contrary to what Dryden had been quoted as saying in the *OED*—that *protagonist* is a word that can only ever be used in the singular.

Any use suggesting the contrary would be grammatically utterly wrong. And not just wrong, Fowler declares, but absurd. It would be nonsense to suggest that there could ever be two characters in a play, both of whom could be described as the most important. One either is the most important person, or one is not.

It took more than half a century before the *OED* decided to settle the matter. The 1981 *Supplement*, in the classically magisterial way of the dictionary, tries to counter the excitable (and now, as it happens, late, Mr. Fowler). It offers a new quotation, reinforcing the view that the word can be used plurally or singularly as the need arises. George Bernard Shaw, it says, wrote in 1950: "Living actors have to learn that they too must be invisible while the protagonists are conversing, and therefore must not move a muscle nor change their expression." Perhaps Fowler's great linguistic authority was technically correct but, the dictionary explains in an expanded version of its 1928 definition, perhaps only in the specific terms of classical Greek theater for which the word was first devised.

In the commonsense world of modern English—the world that, after all, the great dictionary was designed to reify and define—to fix, in dictionary-speak—it is surely quite reasonable to have two or more leading players in any story. Many dramas have room for more than one hero, and both or all may be equally heroic. If the ancient Greeks were one-hero dramatists, then so be it. In the rest of the world, there could be as many as the dramatists cared to write parts for.

Now there is a twenty-volume second edition of the dictionary, with all the material from the supplements fully integrated with the original work, and new words and forms that have emerged in the years since inserted as needs be. In that edition *protagonist* appears in what is currently considered to be its true fixity: with three main meanings and nineteen supporting quotations. Dryden's remains unaltered, the first appearance of the word, *and* in the plural; and to give even greater weight to the notion that the plural is a perfectly acceptable form, both *The Times* and the thriller writer and medievalist Dorothy L. Sayers are quoted in addition to Shaw. The word is thus now properly lexically set for all time, and is stated by the almost unchallengeable authority of the *OED* to be available for use in either the singular or the multiple.

Which happens to be just as well, considering—and to reiterate the point—the existence of two protagonists in this story.

The first one, as is already clear, is Dr. William Chester Minor, the admitted and insane American murderer. The other is a man whose lifetime was more or less coincident with Minor's, but who was different in almost all its other respects: He was named James Augustus Henry Murray. The lives of the two men were over the years to become inextricably and most curiously entwined.

And, moreover, both were to be entwined with the *Oxford English Dictionary,* since the second of the two men, James Murray, was to become for the last forty years of his life its greatest and most justly famous editor.

James Murray was born in February 1837, the eldest son of a tailor and linen draper in Hawick, a pretty little market town in the valley of the Teviot River, in the Scottish Borders. And that was about all that he really wished the world to know about himself. "I am a nobody," he would write toward the end of the century, when fame had begun to creep up on him. "Treat me as a solar myth, or an echo, or an irrational quantity, or ignore me altogether."

But it has long since proved impossible to ignore him, as he was to become a towering figure in British scholarship. Honors were showered on him during his lifetime, and he has achieved the standing of a mythic hero since his death. Murray's childhood alone, which was uncovered twenty years ago by his granddaughter Elisabeth, who opened his trunk of papers, hints temptingly that he was destined—despite his unpromising, unmoneyed, unsophisticated beginnings—for extraordinary things.

He was a precocious, very serious little boy; he turned steadily into an astonishingly learned teenager, tall, well built, with long hair and an early, bright red beard that added to his grave and forbidding appearance. "Knowledge is power," he declared on the flyleaf of his school exercise book, and added—for as well as having a working knowledge by the time he was fifteen of French, Italian, German, and Greek, he, like all educated children then, knew Latin— "*Nihil est melius quam vita diligentissima*" (Nothing is better than a most diligent life).

He had a voracious appetite, indeed an impassioned thirst for all kinds of learning. He taught himself about the local geology and botany; he found a globe from which he could learn geography and foster a love for maps; he unearthed scores of textbooks from which he could take on the enormous burden of history; he observed and took pains to remember all the natural phenomena about him. His younger brothers would tell how he once awakened them late one night to show them the rising of Sirius, the Dog Star, whose orbit and appearance over the horizon he had calculated and that proved, to the family's sleepy exultation, to be perfectly correct.

He particularly cherished encountering and interrogating people he met who proved to be living links with history: He once found an ancient who had known someone who was present when Parliament proclaimed William and Mary joint sovereigns in 1689; then again, his mother would recount over and over how she had heard tell of the victory at Waterloo; and when he had children himself he would allow them to be dandled on the knees of an elderly naval officer who was present when Napoleon agreed to surrender.

He left school at fourteen, as did most of the poorer children of the British Isles. There was no money for him to go on to the fee-paying grammar school in nearby Melrose, and in any case his parents enjoyed some confidence in the lad's ability to teach himself—by pursuing, as he had vowed, the *vita diligentissima*. Their hopes proved well founded: James continued to amass more and more knowledge, if only (as he would admit) for the sake of knowledge itself, and often in the most eccentric of ways.

He engaged in furious digs at a multitude of archaeological sites all over the Borders (which, being close to Hadrian's Wall, was a treasure trove of buried antiquities); he made attempts to teach the local cows to respond to calls in Latin; he would read out loud, by the light of a minute oil lamp, the works of a Frenchman with the grand name of Théodore Agrippa d'Aubigné, and translating for his family, who gathered about him, fascinated.

Once, trying to invent water wings made from bundles of pond iris, he tied them to his arms but was turned upside down by more buoyancy than he calculated, and would have drowned (he was a nonswimmer) had not his friends rescued him by pulling him from the lake with his five-foot-long bow tie. He memorized hundreds of phrases in Romany, the language of the passing Gypsies; he learned bookbinding; he taught himself to embellish his own writings with elegant little drawings, flourishes, and curlicues, rather like the monkish illuminators of the Middle Ages.

By seventeen this "argumentative, earnest, naïve" young Scot was employed in his hometown, as an assistant head-master, eagerly passing on the knowledge that he had so keenly amassed; by twenty he was a full-fledged headmaster of the local subscription academy ("ages ten to sixteen, fees one guinea a term"); and with his brother Alexander he be-came a leading member of that most Victorian and Scottish of bodies, the Hawick branch of the Mutual Improvement Institute. He gave his first lecture—"Reading, Its Pleasures and Advantages"—and went on to present learned papers to the town's Literary and Philosophical Society on his new pas-sion of phonetics, on the origins of the pronunciation and the foundations of the Scottish tongue, and—once he had discov-ered its delights—on the magic of Anglo-Saxon.

And yet all this early promise seemed suddenly doomed, first by the onset of love and then by the upset of tragedy. For in 1861, when he was just twenty-four, James met and the fol-lowing year married a handsome but delicate infant-school music teacher named Maggie Scott. Their wedding picture shows James a strangely tall, vaguely simian figure in his ill-fitting frock coat and baggy trousers; a man with hugely long, knee-brushing arms; an unkempt beard; hair already thin-ning near the peak; eyes narrow and intense: neither happy nor unhappy, but full of thought, his mind seemingly filled with a kind of distracted foreboding.

Two years later they had a baby girl they christened Anna. But, as was wretchedly commonplace at the time, she died in infancy. Maggie Murray herself then fell gravely ill with consumption and was said by the Hawick doctors to be unlikely to withstand the rigors of another long Scottish winter. The recommended treatment was to sojourn in the South of France but that, given James's tiny schoolmastering wage, was quite out of the question.

Instead the forlorn couple took off for London and modest lodgings in Peckham. James Murray, now twenty-seven, had to his bitter disappointment been forced by his domestic circumstances to abandon all his current intellectual pursuits, all his digging and delving and his pronouncements on linguistics, phonetics, and the origins of words—on which topic he was then enjoying a lively correspondence with the notable scholar Alexander Melville Bell, father of the infinitely more famous Alexander Graham Bell.

Economic necessity and marital duty—though he was devoted to Maggie and never complained—had pressed him to become instead, and with a dreary predictability, a clerk in a London bank. With his employment, in starched cuffs and green eyeshade, perched on a high stool at the back of the head office of the Chartered Bank of India, it seemed as though the story might have come to an ignominious end.

Not so. Within just a matter of months he was back in the traces. He had renewed his eccentric pursuit of learning—studying Hindustani and Achaemenid Persian on his daily commute, trying to determine by their accents from which region of Scotland various London policemen came, lecturing on "The Body and its Architecture" before the Camberwell Congregational Church (where, as a confirmed and lifelong teetotaler, he was a keen member of the Temperance League), and even noting with amused detachment, while his still-sickly and well-loved Maggie was dying, that in her nightly delirium she lapsed into the broad Scots dialect of her childhood, abandoning the more refined tones of a schoolteacher. That small discovery, that marginal addition to his learning, went some way to helping him through the misery of her subsequent death.

A year later James was engaged to another young woman and a year later still, married. While he had clearly loved and admired Maggie Scott, it was soon abundantly clear that in Ada Ruthven, whose father worked for the Great Indian Peninsular Railway and was an admirer of Alexander von Humboldt, and whose mother claimed to have been at school with Charlotte Brontë, here was a woman who was far more his social and intellectual equal. They were to remain devoted, and to have eleven children together, the first nine, according to the wishes of James's father-in-law, bearing the middle name Ruthven.

A letter that James Murray wrote in 1867, his thirtieth year, applying for a position with the British Museum, offers some of the flavor of his barely believable range of knowledge (as well as his unabashed candor in telling people about it):

> I have to state that Philology, both Comparative and special, has been my favourite pursuit during the whole of my life, and that I possess a general acquaintance with the languages & literature of the

Aryan and Syro-Arabic classes—not indeed to say that I am familiar with all or nearly all of these, but that I possess that general lexical and structural knowledge which makes the intimate knowledge only a matter of a little application. With several I have a more intimate acquaintance as with the Romance tongues, Italian, French, Catalan, Spanish, Latin & in a less degree Portuguese, Vaudois, Provençal and various dialects. In the Teutonic branch, I am tolerably familiar with Dutch (having at my place of business correspondence to read in Dutch, German, French & occasionally other languages), Flemish, German, Danish. In Anglo-Saxon and Moeso-Gothic my studies have been much closer, I having prepared some works for publication upon these languages. I know a little of the Celtic, and am at present engaged with the Sclavonic, having obtained a useful knowledge of the Russian. In the Persian, Achaemenian Cuneiform, & Sanscrit branches, I know for the purposes of Comparative Philology. I have sufficient knowledge of Hebrew and Syriac to read at sight the Old Testament and Peshito; to a less degree I know Aramaic Arabic, Coptic and Phoenician to the point where it was left by Genesius.

It somewhat beggars belief that the museum turned his job application down. Murray was initially crushed but soon recovered. Before long he was consoling himself in a characteristic way—by comparing, in lexical terms, the sheep-counting numerology of the Wowenoc Indians of Maine with that of the moorland farmers of Yorkshire.

Murray's interest in philology might have remained that of an enthusiastic amateur had it not been for his friendship with two men. One was a Trinity College, Cambridge, mathematician named Alexander Ellis, and the other a notoriously pigheaded, colossally rude phonetician named Henry Sweet—the figure on whom Bernard Shaw would later base his character Professor Henry Higgins in *Pygmalion*, which was transmuted later into the eternally popular *My Fair Lady* (in which Higgins was played, in the film, by the similarly rude and pigheaded actor Rex Harrison).

These men swiftly turned the amateur dabbler and dilettante into a serious philological scholar. Murray was introduced into membership of the august and exclusive Philological Society—no mean achievement for a young man who, it must be recalled, had left school at fourteen and had not thus far attended a university. By 1869 he was on the society's council. In 1873—having left the bank and gone back to teaching (at Mill Hill School)—he published *The Dialect of the Southern Counties of Scotland*: It was a work that was to gild and solidify his reputation to the point of wide admiration (and to win him the invitation to contribute an essay on the history of the English language for the ninth edition of the *Encyclopædia Britannica*). It also brought him into contact with one of the most amazing men of Victorian England—the half-mad scholar-gypsy who was secretary of the Philological Society, Frederick Furnivall.

Some thought Furnivall—despite his devotion to mathematics, Middle English, and philology—a total clown, an ass, a scandalous dandy, and a fool (his critics, who were legion, made much of the fact that his father maintained a private lunatic asylum in the house where the young Frederick had grown up).

He was a socialist, an agnostic, and a vegetarian, and "to alcohol and tobacco he was a stranger all his life." He was a keen athlete, obsessed by sculling, and was particularly fond of teaching handsome young waitresses (recruited from the ABC teashop in New Oxford Street) the best way to get the most speed out of a slender racing boat he had designed. A photograph of him survives from 1901: He wears an impish smirk, not least because he is surrounded by eight pretty members of the Hammersmith Sculling Club for Girls, content and well-exercised women whose skirts may be long but whose shirts lie snug on their ample breasts. In the background stands a stern Victorian matron, clad all in tough serge weeds, scowling.

Frederick Furnivall was indeed an appalling flirt. He was condemned by many as socially reprehensible for committing the doubly unpardonable sin of marrying a lady's maid and then abandoning her. Dozens of editors and publishers refused to work with him: he was "devoid of tact or discretion . . . had a boyish frankness of speech which offended many and led him into unedifying controversies . . . his declarations of hostility to religion and to class distinctions were often unreasonable and gave pain."

But he was a brilliant scholar, and, like James Murray,

he had an obsessive thirst for learning; among his friends and admirers he could count Alfred, Lord Tennyson; Charles Kingsley; William Morris; John Ruskin—Doctor Minor's London mentor, it would later turn out—and the Yorkshire-born composer Frederick Delius. Kenneth Grahame, a fellow sculler who worked at the Bank of England, came duly under Furnivall's spell, wrote *The Wind in the Willows* and painted Furnivall into the plot as the Water Rat. "We learned em!" says Toad. "We taught em" corrects Rat. Furnivall may have been a cunning mischief-maker, but he was also often right.

He may have been Grahame's mentor; but he was a much more significant figure in James Murray's life. As the latter's biographer was to say, admiringly, Furnivall was to Murray "stimulating and persuasive, often meddlesome and exasperating, always a dynamic and powerful influence, eclipsing even James in his gusto for life."

He was in many ways a Victorian's Victorian, an Englishman's Englishman—and a natural choice, as the country's leading philologist, to take a dominant role in the making of the great new dictionary that was then in the process of being constructed.

It was Furnivall's friendship with and sponsorship of James Murray—as well as Murray's links with Sweet and Ellis—that were to lead, ultimately, to the most satisfactory event of all. This occurred on the afternoon of April 26, 1878, at which time James Augustus Henry Murray was invited to Oxford, to a room in Christ Church College, Oxford, and to an awesome full meeting of the grandest minds in the land, the Delegates of the Oxford University Press.

They were a formidable group—the college dean, Henry Liddell (whose daughter Alice had so captivated the Christ Church mathematician Charles Lutwidge Dodgson that he wrote an adventure book for her, set in Wonderland); Max Müller, the Leipzig philologist, Orientalist, and Sanskrit scholar who now held Oxford's chair of Comparative Philology; the Regius Professor of History, William Stubbs, the man who was credited in Victorian times with having made the subject worthy of respectable academic pursuit; the canon of Christ Church and classical scholar, Edwin Palmer; the warden of New College, James Sewell—and so on and so on.

High Church, high learning, high ambition: These were the Men Who Counted, the architects of the great intellectual constructions that originated during England's haughtiest and most self-confident time. As Isambard Kingdom Brunel was to bridges and railways, as Sir Richard Burton was to Africa, and as Robert Falcon Scott was soon to be to the Antarctic, so these men were the best, the makers of indelible monuments to learning—of the books that were to be the core foundation of the great libraries all around the globe.

And they had a project, they said, in which Doctor Murray might well be very interested indeed. A project that, unwittingly on the parts of all concerned, was eventually to put James Murray on a collision course with a man whose interests and whose piety were curiously congruent with his own.

*   *   *

At first blush William Minor might seem to have been a man more marked by his differences from Murray than by such similarities as these. He was rich where Murray was poor. He was of high estate where Murray's condition was irredeemably, if respectably, low. And though he was almost the same age—just three years separated them—he had been born both of a different citizenship and, as it happens, in a place that was almost as many thousands of miles away from Murray's British Isles as it was then thought prudent and practicable for ordinary people to reach.

3

The Madness of War

Lunatic (lˈū nătik), *a.* [ad. late L. *lūnātic-us*, f. L. *lūna* moon: see -ATIC. Cf. F. *lunatique*, Sp., It. *lunatico*.] **A.** *adj.*

   1. Originally, affected with the kind of insanity that was supposed to have recurring periods dependent on the changes of the moon. In mod. use, synonymous with INSANE; current in popular and legal language, but not now employed technically by physicians.

Ceylon, the lushly overgrown tropical island that seems to hang from India's southern tip like a teardrop—or a pear or a pearl or even (some say) a Virginia ham—is regarded by priests of the world's stricter religions as the place to which Adam and Eve were exiled after their fall from grace. It is a Garden of Eden for sinners, an island limbo for those who yielded to temptation.

These days it is called Sri Lanka; once the Arab sea traders called it Serendib, and in the eighteenth century Horace Walpole created a fanciful story about three princes who reigned there, and who had the enchanting habit of stumbling across wonderful things quite by chance. Thus was the English language enriched by the word *serendipity*, without its inventor, who never traveled to the East, ever really knowing why.

But as it happens Walpole was more accurate than he could ever have known. Ceylon is in reality a kind of postlapsarian treasure island, where every sensual gift of the tropics is available, both to reward temptation and to beguile and charm. So there are cinnamon and coconut, coffee and tea; there are sapphires and rubies, mangoes and cashews, elephants and leopards; and everywhere a rich, hot, sweetly moist breeze, scented by the sea, spices, and blossoms.

And there are the girls—young, chocolate-skinned, ever-giggling naked girls with sleek wet bodies, rosebud nipples, long hair, coltish legs, and scarlet and purple petals folded behind their ears—who play in the white Indian Ocean surf and who run, quite without shame, along the cool wet sands on their way back home.

It was these nameless village girls—the likes of whom had frolicked naked in the Singhalese surf for scores of years past, just as they still do—that young William Chester Minor remembered most. It was these young girls of Ceylon, he later said he was sure, who had unknowingly set him on the spiral path to his eventually insatiable lust, to his incurable madness, and to his final perdition. He had first noticed the erotic thrill of their charms when he was just thirteen years old: It was to inflame a shaming obsession with sexuality that inspired his senses and sapped his energies from that moment on.

William Minor was born on the island in June 1834—a little more than three years before, and fully five thousand miles to the east of, James Murray, the man with whom he would soon become so inextricably linked. And in one respect—and one only—the lives of the two so widely separated families were similar: Both the Murrays and the Minors were exceedingly pious.

Thomas and Mary Murray were members of the Congregationalist Church, clinging to the conservative ways of seventeenth-century Scotland with a group known as the Covenanters. Eastman and Lucy Minor were Congregationalists too, but of the more muscularly evangelical kind that dominated the American colonies, and whose views and beliefs were descended from those of the Pilgrim Fathers. And although Eastman Strong Minor had learned the skills of printing, and had prospered as the owner of a press, his life eventually became devoted to taking the light of homespun American Protestantism into the dark interiors of the East Indies. The Minors were in Ceylon as missionaries, and when William was born it was at the mission clinic, into a devout mission family.

Unlike the Murrays, the Minors were first-line American aristocracy. The original settler in the New World was

Thomas Minor, who came originally from the village of Chew Magna in Gloucestershire. He had sailed across the Atlantic less than a decade after the Pilgrims, aboard a ship called the *Lion's Whelp*, which landed at Stonington, the port beside Mystic, at the mouth of Long Island Sound. Of the nine children born to Thomas and his wife, Grace, six were boys, all of whom went on to spread the family name throughout New England, and be counted among the devout and high-principled founding fathers of the state of Connecticut in the late seventeenth century.

Eastman Strong Minor, who was born in Milford in 1809, was the head of the seventh generation of American Minors; the family members were by now generally prosperous, settled, respected. Few thought it other than a badge of honor when Eastman and his young Bostonian wife, Lucy, whom he married in her city in 1833, closed down the family printshop and took off by steamer carrying a cargo of ice from Salem for Ceylon. Their piety was well known, and the Minor family seemed delighted that, in spite of the couple's wealth and social standing, they felt strongly enough in their calling to contemplate spending what would probably be many years away from the United States, preaching the gospel to those regarded as less fortunate far away.

They arrived in Ceylon in March 1834, and were settled in the mission station in a village called Manepay, on the island's northeast coast, close to the great British naval station at Trincomalee. It was only three months later, in June, that William was born—his mother having suffered badly through the addition of seasickness to morning sickness during the middle of her pregnancy. A second child, named Lucy, like her mother, was born two years later.

Although William's medical file suggests a typically rugged Indian childhood—breaking a collarbone in a fall from a horse, being knocked unconscious after falling from a tree, the usual slight doses of malaria and blackwater fever—his was far from a normal childhood.

His mother died of consumption when he was three. Two years later, instead of returning home to the United States with his two young children, Eastman Minor set off on a journey through the Malay Peninsula, bent on finding a second wife among the mission communities there. He left his little girl in charge of a pair of missionaries in a Singhalese village called Oodooville and took off on an eastbound tramp steamer with young William in tow.

The pair arrived in Singapore, where Minor had a mutual friend who introduced him to a party of American missionaries bound upcountry to preach the gospels in Bangkok. One of them was a handsome (and conveniently orphaned) divine named Judith Manchester Taylor, who came from Madison, New York. They courted quickly, and tactfully out of sight of the curious child who had accompanied them. Minor persuaded Miss Taylor to come back with them on the next Jaffna-bound steamer, and they were married by the American consul in Colombo shortly before Christmas 1839.

Judith Minor was as energetic as her printer husband. She ran the local school, learned Singhalese, and taught it to her clearly very intelligent elder stepchild as well as, in due course, to her own six children.

Two of the sons that resulted from this marriage died, the first aged one, the second five. One of William's stepsisters died when she was eight. His own sister, Lucy, died of consumption when she was twenty-one. (A third half-brother, Thomas T. Minor, died in peculiar circumstances many years later. He moved to the American West, first as doctor to the Winnebago tribe in Nebraska, then to the newly acquired Alaskan Territory to collect specimens of Arctic habitations, and finally on to Port Townsend and Seattle, where he was elected mayor. In 1889, still holding the post, he took off on a canoe expedition to Whidbey Island with a friend, G. Morris Haller. Neither man ever returned. Neither boats nor bodies were ever found. A Minor Street and a Thomas T. Minor School remain, as well as a reputation in Seattle that equates the name of Minor with some degree of glamour, pioneering, and mystery.)

The mission library at Manepay was well stocked, and though the accommodation for the family was "very poor," according to Judith's diaries, the mission school itself was excellent—allowing young William to win a markedly better education than he might have received back in New England. His father's printing tasks gave him access to literature and newspapers; and his parents traveled by horse and buggy often, taking him along and encouraging him to learn as many of the local languages as possible. By the time he was twelve he spoke good Singhalese and is supposed to have had a fair grounding in Burmese, as well as some Hindi and Tamil, and a smattering of various Chinese dialects. He also knew his way around Singapore, Bangkok, and Rangoon, as well as the island of Penang, off the coast of what was then British Malaya.

William was just thirteen, he later told his doctors, when he first started to enjoy "lascivious thoughts" about the young Ceylonese girls on the sands around him: they must have seemed a rare constant in a shifting, inconstant life. But by the time he was fourteen, his parents (who were perhaps aware of his pubescent longings) decided to send him back to the United States, well away from the temptations of the tropics. He was to live with his uncle Alfred, who then ran a large crockery shop in the center of New Haven. So William was seen off from the port of Colombo on one of the regular P & O liners that made the unendurably lengthy passage between Bombay and London—via (this being in 1848, long before the completion of the Suez Canal) the long seas around the Cape of Good Hope.

He later admitted to vividly erotic recollections from the voyage. In particular he remembered being "fiercely attracted" to a young English girl he met aboard ship. He seems not to have been warned that long tropical days and nights at sea—combined with the slow, rocking motion of the swell and the tendency for women to wear short, light cotton dresses and for bartenders to offer exotic drinks—could very well, in those days as well as these, lead to romance, particularly when one or even both sets of parents were absent.

Much appears to have happened during the four weeks at sea—though not, perhaps, the ultimate. The friendship appears to have gone unconsummated, no matter how much time the pair spent alone. Many years later Minor was to point out to his doctors that, as with his fantasies over the young Indian girls, he never "gratified himself in an unnatural way" or ever let his sexual feelings for his fellow passenger get the better of him. Matters might have turned out very differently if they had.

Guilt—perhaps a frequent handmaiden among the peculiarly pious—seems to have intervened, even more than a teenager's shyness or natural caution. From this moment on in William Minor's long and tormented life, sex and guilt come to appear firmly and fatally riveted together. He keeps apologizing to his questioners of later years: His thoughts were "lascivious," he was "ashamed" of them, he did his best not to "yield" to them. He seems to have been looking over his shoulder all the time, making sure that his parents—perhaps the mother whom he lost when he was barely out of infancy, or perhaps the stepmother, so often the cause of problems for male children—never came to know the "vile machinations," as he saw them, of his increasingly troubled mind.

But these feelings were still nascent in William Minor's teenage years, and at the time he was unworried by them. He had his academic life to pursue, and eagerly. From London he took another ship to Boston, and thence home to New Haven, where he began the arduous task of studying medicine at Yale University. His parents and their much-diminished family were not to return for six more years, by which time he was twenty. He appears to have spent these—and indeed the following nine years of his medical apprenticeship—in quietly assiduous study, setting to one side what would soon become his deeper concerns.

He passed all his examinations without any apparent undue problems and was graduated by the Yale Medical School with a degree and a specialization in comparative anatomy in February 1863, when he was twenty-nine. The only recorded drama of those years came when he caught a serious infection after cutting his hand while conducting a postmortem on a man who had died of septicemia: He reacted quickly, painting his hand with iodine—but not quickly enough. He had been gravely ill, his doctors later said, and had nearly died.

By now he was a grown man, tempered by his years in the East and honed by his studies at what was already one of the finest American schools. Although he had no inkling that his mind was in so perilously fragile a state, he was about to embark on what was almost certainly the most traumatic period of his young life. He applied to join the army as a surgeon—an army that at the time was keenly short of medical personnel. For it was not just the army—it was then calling itself the Union army: The United States, still young also, was just then suffering the most traumatic period of its national life. The Civil War was well under way.

When Minor signed his first contract with the army—which first trained him conveniently close to home at the Knight Hospital in New Haven—the war was almost precisely half-way over, though naturally none knew this at the time. Eight hundred days of it had been fought so far: Men had seen the Battles of Forts Sumter, Clark, Hatteras, and Henry; the First

and Second Battles of Bull Run; and the fights over patches
of land at Chancellorsville, Fredericksburg, Vicksburg, An-
tietam, and scores of otherwise unsung and unremembered
trophies, like Mississippi's Big Black River Bridge, or Island
Number Ten, Missouri, or Greasy Creek, Kentucky. The
South had so far had an abundance of victories: The Union
Army, sorely pressed by eight hundred days of bitter fighting
and far too many reverses, would take all the men it could:
It was eager to accept someone as apparently competent and
well-Yankee-born as William Chester Minor of Yale.

Four days after he joined up, on June 29, 1863, came
the Battle of Gettysburg, the bloodiest of the entire war, the
turning point, beyond which the Confederacy's military ambitions began to fail. The newspapers that Minor read each
evening in New Haven were full of accounts of the progress
of the fighting; there were twenty thousand casualties on the
Union side, and to those numbers even a tiny state like Connecticut contributed a monstrous share—it lost more than a
quarter of the men it sent to fight in Pennsylvania over those
three July days. The world, President Lincoln was to say six
months later when he consecrated the land as a memorial to
the fallen, could never forget what they had done there.

No doubt the tales of the battle stirred the young surgeon:
There were casualties aplenty out there, abundant work for
an energetic and ambitious young doctor to do, and besides,
he was on what now looked very much like the winning side.
By August he was fully sworn in to do the army's bidding; by
November he was under formal contract to serve as an acting assistant surgeon, to do whatever the Surgeon General's

Department demanded. He was itching, his brother was to testify later, to be sent to the seat of battle.

But it was six more months before the army finally agreed and transferred him down south, close to the sounds of war. In New Haven he had spent a relatively easy time, taking care of men who had been brought far away from the trauma of fighting, men who were now healing, both in body and mind. But down in northern Virginia where he was first sent, all was very different.

There the full horror of this cruel and fearsomely bloody struggle came home to him, suddenly, without warning. Here was an inescapable irony of the Civil War, not known in any conflict between men before or since: the fact that this was a war fought with new and highly effective weapons, machines for the mowing down of men—and yet at a time when an era of poor and primitive medicine was just coming to an end. It was fought with the mortar and the musket and the minié ball, but not yet quite with anesthesia or with sulphonamides and penicillin. The common soldier was thus in a poorer position than at any time before: He could be monstrously ill treated by all the new weaponry, and yet only moderately well treated with all the old medicine.

So in the field hospitals there was gangrene, amputation, filth, pain, and disease—the appearance of pus in a wound was said by doctors to be "laudable," the sign of healing. The sounds in the first-aid tents were unforgettable: the screams and whimperings of men whose lives had been ruined by cruel new guns and in ferocious and ceaseless battles. Some 360,000 Federal troops died in the war, and so did 258,000

Confederates—and for every one who died of wounds caused by the new weapons, so two died from incidental infection, illness, and poor hygiene.

To Minor this was all still terribly alien. He was, his friends at home would later say, a sensitive man—courteous to a fault, somewhat academic, rather too gentle for the business of soldiering. He read, painted watercolors, played the flute. But Virginia in 1864 was no place for the genteel and mild mannered. And although it is never quite possible to pinpoint what causes the eruption of madness in a man, there is at least some circumstantial suggestion in this case that it was an event, or a coincidence of events, that finally did unhinge Doctor Minor and pitch him over the edge into what in those unforgiving times was regarded as total lunacy.

Given what we now know about the setting and the circumstance of his first encounter with war, it does seem at least reasonable and credible to suppose that his madness—latent, hovering in the background—was triggered at that time. Something specific seems to have happened in Orange County, Virginia, early in May 1864, during the two days of the astonishingly bloody encounter that has since come to be called the Battle of the Wilderness. It was a fight to test the sanest of men: Some of the occurrences of those two days were utterly beyond human imagination.

It is not clear exactly why Minor went to the Wilderness—his written orders in fact called for him to proceed from New Haven to Washington and to the medical director's office, where he would replace a Doctor Abbott, then working at an army divisional hospital in Alexandria. He eventually did as he was bidden—but first, and possibly on the specific orders of the medical director—he went eighty miles to the southwest of the Federal capital into the field, where he would see—for the first and only time in his career—real fighting.

The Battle of the Wilderness was the first genuine working test of the assumption that, with the Gettysburg victory in July 1863, the tide of events in the Civil War truly had changed. The following March, President Lincoln had placed all Union forces under the command of Gen. Ulysses S. Grant, who swiftly devised a master plan that called for nothing less than the total destruction of the Confederate armies. The scattershot and ill-organized campaigns of the weeks and months before—skirmishes here and there, towns and forts captured and recaptured—meant nothing in terms of coherent strategy: So long as the Confederate army remained intact and ready to fight, so Jefferson Davis's Confederacy remained. Kill the secessionist army, Grant reasoned, and you kill the secessionist cause.

This grand strategy got formally under way in May 1864, when the great military machine that Grant had assembled for finishing off the Confederate army began to roll southward from the Potomac. The campaign triggered by this first sweep would eventually cut through Dixie like a scythe; Sherman would rage from Tennessee through Georgia, Savannah would be captured, the main Confederate forces would surrender at Appomattox a mere eleven months later, and the final fight of the five-year war would take place in Louisiana, at Shreveport, almost a year to the day after Grant began to move.

But the beginnings of the strategy were the most difficult to execute, with the enemy at its least broken and most determined—and rarely in those early weeks was the battle more fiercely joined than on the campaign's first day. General Grant's men marched along the foothills of the Blue Ridge Mountains and, on the afternoon of May 4, crossed the Rapidan River into Orange County. There they met Robert E. Lee's Army of Northern Virginia: The subsequent fight, which began with the river crossing and ended only when Grant's men made a flanking pass out toward Spotsylvania, cost some twenty-seven thousand lives in just fifty hours of savagery and fire.

Three distinct aspects of this enormous battle appear to make it particularly important in the story of Dr. William Minor.

The first was the sheer and savage ferocity of the engagement and the pitiless conditions on the field where it was fought. The thousands of men who faced each other did so in a landscape that was utterly unsuited for infantry tactics. It was—and still is—a gently sloping kind of countryside, thickly covered with second-growth timber and impenetrably dense underbrush. There are tracts of swamp country, muddy and fetid, heavy with mosquitoes. In May it is dreadfully hot, and the foliage away from the swamps and seeping brooks is always tinder dry.

The fighting therefore was conducted not with artillery—

which couldn't see—nor with cavalry—which couldn't ride. It had to be conducted by infantrymen with muskets—their guns charged with the dreadful flesh-tearing minié ball, a newfangled kind of bullet that was expanded by a powder charge in its base and inflicted huge, unsightly wounds—or hand-to-hand, with bayonets and sabers. And with the heat and smoke of battle came yet another terror—fire.

The brush caught ablaze, and flames tore through the wilderness ahead of a stiff, hot wind. Hundreds, perhaps thousands of men, the wounded as well as the fit, were burned to death, suffering the most terrible agonies.

One doctor wrote how soldiers appeared to have been wounded "in every conceivable way, men with mutilated bodies, with shattered limbs and broken heads, men enduring their injuries with stoic patience, and men giving way to violent grief, men stoically indifferent, and men bravely rejoicing that—it is only a leg!" Such tracks as existed were jammed with crude wagons pulling blood-soaked casualties to the dressing stations, where overworked, sweating doctors tried their best to deal with injuries of the most gruesome kind.

A soldier from Maine wrote with appalled wonder of the fire. "The blaze ran sparkling and crackling up the trunks of the pines, till they stood a pillar of fire from base to topmost spray. Then they wavered and fell, throwing up showers of gleaming sparks, while over all hung the thick clouds of dark smoke, reddened beneath by the glare of flames."

"Forest fires raged," wrote another soldier who was at the Wilderness,

ammunition trains exploded; the dead were roasted
in the conflagration; the wounded, roused by its hot
breath, dragged themselves along with their torn
and mangled limbs, in the mad energy of despair,
to escape the ravages of the flames; and every bush
seemed hung with shreds of bloodstained clothing.
It seemed as though Christian men had turned to
fiends, and hell itself had usurped the place of earth.

The second aspect of the battle that may be important in
understanding Minor's bewildering pathology relates to one
particular group who played a part in the fighting: the Irish.
The same Irish of whom Minor's London landlady would
later testify that he appeared to be strangely frightened.

There were around 150,000 Irish soldiers on the Union
side in the struggle, many of them subsumed anonymously
into the Yankee units that happened to recruit where they
lived. But there was also a proud assemblage of Irishmen
who fought together, as a block: These were the soldiers of the
Second Brigade—the Irish Brigade—and they were braver
and rougher than almost any other unit in the entire Federal
army. "When anything absurd, forlorn, or desperate was to
be attempted," as one English war correspondent wrote, "the
Irish Brigade was called upon."

The brigade fought at the Wilderness: Men of the 28th
Massachusetts and the 116th Pennsylvania were there, alongside Irishmen from New York's legendary regiments, the
63rd, the 88th, and the 69th—which still, to this day, leads

the Saint Patrick's Day parade up the green-lined expanse of
Fifth Avenue in March.

But compared with those who had fought one or two
years before, there was a subtle difference in the mood of the
Irishmen who fought with the Federal troops in 1864. At the
beginning of the war, before Emancipation had been proclaimed, the Irish were staunch in their support of the North,
and equally antipathetic to a South that seemed, at least in
those early days, to be backed by the England they so loathed.
Their motives in fighting were complex—but once again it is
a complexity that is important to this story. They were new
immigrants from a famine-racked Ireland, and they were
fighting in America not just out of gratitude to a country that
had given them succor but in order to be trained to fight back
home one day, and to rid their island of the hated English
once and for all. An Irish-American poem of the time made
the point:

> When concord and peace to this land are restored,
> And the union's established for ever,
> Brave sons of Hibernia, oh, sheathe not the sword;—
> You will then have a union to sever.

The Irish were not to remain long in sympathy with all
of the Federal aims. They were fierce rivals with American
blacks, competing at the base of the social ladder for such
opportunities—work, especially—as were on offer. And once
the slaves were formally emancipated by Lincoln in 1863,

the natural advantage that the Irish believed they had in the color of their skins quite vanished—and with it much of their sympathy for the Union cause in the war they had chosen to fight. Besides, they had been doing their sums: "We did not cause this war," one of their leaders said, "but vast numbers of our people have perished for it."

The consequence was that—especially in battles where it seemed as though the Irish troops were being used as cannon fodder—they began to leave the fields of battle. They began to run away, to desert. And large numbers of them certainly deserted from the terrible flames and bloodshed of the Battle of the Wilderness. It was desertion, and one of the particular punishments often inflicted on those convicted of it, that stands as the third and possibly the principal reason for William Minor's subsequent fall.

Desertion, like indiscipline and drunkenness, was a chronic problem during the Civil War—seriously so because it deprived the commanders of the manpower they so badly needed. It was a problem that grew as the war itself endured—the enthusiasm of the two causes abating as the months and years went on and the numbers of casualties grew. The total strength of the Union army was probably 2,900,000, and that of the Confederacy 1,300,000—and as we have seen, they suffered staggering casualty totals of 360,000 and 258,000 respectively. The number of men who simply dropped their guns and fled into the forest is almost equally spectacular—287,000 from the Union side, 103,000 from the Southern states. Of course these figures are somewhat distorted: They represent men who fled, were captured, and set to fighting again, only to desert once more and maybe many times subsequently. But they are still gigantic numbers—one in ten in the Union army, one in twelve from the rebels.

By the middle of the war more than five thousand soldiers were deserting every month—some merely dropping behind during the interminable route marches, others fleeing in the face of gunfire. In May 1864—the month when General Grant began his southern progress, and the month of the Wilderness—no fewer than 5,371 Federal soldiers cut and ran. More than 170 left the field every day—they were both draftees and volunteers, and either heartsick or homesick, depressed, bored, disillusioned, unpaid, or just plain scared. William Minor had not merely stumbled from the calm of Connecticut into a scene of carnage and horror: He had also come across a demonstration of man at his least impressive— fearful, depleted in spirit, and cowardly.

Army regulations of the time may have been rather flexible when it came to prescribing penalties for drinking—a common punishment was to make the man stand on a box for several days, with a billet of wood on his shoulder—but they were unambiguous when it came to desertion. Anyone caught and convicted of "the one sin which may not be pardoned in this world or the next" would be shot. That, at least, was what was said on paper: "Desertion is a crime punishable by death."

But to shoot one of your own soldiers, whatever his crime, had a practical disbenefit—it diminished your own numbers, weakened your own forces. This piece of grimly realistic arithmetic persuaded most Civil War commanders, on both sides, to devise alternative punishments for those who ran away. Only a couple of hundred men were shot—though their deaths were widely publicized in a vain effort to set an example. Many were thrown into prison, locked in solitary confinement, flogged, or heavily fined.

The rest—and most first-time offenders—were usually subjected to public humiliations of varying kinds. Some had their heads shaved or half shaved, and were forced to wear boards with the inscription "Coward." Some were sentenced by drumhead courts-martial to a painful ordeal called "bucking," in which the wrists were tied tightly, the arms forced over the knees, and a stick secured beneath knees and arms—leaving the convict in an excruciating contortion, often for days at a time. (It was a punishment so harsh as to prove often decidedly counterproductive: One general who ordered a man to be bucked for straggling found that half his company deserted in protest.)

A man could also be gagged with a bayonet, which was tied across his open mouth with twine. He could be suspended from his thumbs, made to carry a yard of rail across his shoulders, be drummed out of town, forced to ride a wooden horse, made to walk around in a barrel shirt and no other clothes—he could even, as in one gruesome case in Tennessee, be nailed to a tree, crucified.

Or else—and here it seemed was the perfect combination of pain and humiliation—he could be branded. The letter *D* would be seared onto his buttock, his hip, or his cheek. It would be a letter one and a half inches high—the regulations became quite specific on this point—and it would either be burned on with a hot iron or cut with a razor and the wound filled with black powder, both to cause irritation and indelibility.

For some unknown reason the regimental drummer boy would often be employed to administer the powder; or in the case of the use of a branding iron, the doctor. And this, it was said at the London trial, was what William Minor had been forced to do.

An Irish deserter, who had been convicted at drumhead of running away during the terrors of the Wilderness, was sentenced to be branded. The officers of the court—there would have been a colonel, four captains, and three lieutenants—demanded in this case that the new young acting assistant surgeon who had been assigned to them, this fresh-faced and genteel-looking aristocrat, this Yalie, fresh down from the hills of New England, be instructed to carry out the punishment. It would be as good a way as any, the old war-weary officers implied, to induct Doctor Minor into the rigors of war. And so the Irishman was brought to him, his arms shackled behind his back.

He was a dirty and unkempt man in his early twenties, his dark uniform torn to rags by his frantic, desperate run through the brambles. He was exhausted and frightened. He was like an animal—a far cry from the young lad who had arrived, cocksure and full of Dublin mischief, on the West Side of Manhattan three years earlier. He had seen so much fighting, so much dying—and yet now the cause for which he had fought was no longer truly his cause, not since Emancipation, certainly. His side was winning, anyway—they wouldn't be needing him anymore, they wouldn't miss him if he ran away.

He wanted to be rid of his duties for the alien Americans. He wanted to go back home to Ireland. He wanted to see his family again and be finished with this strange foreign conflict to which, in truth, he had never been more than a mercenary party. He wanted to use the soldiering skills he had learned in all those fights in Pennsylvania and Maryland and now in the fields of Virginia, to fight against the despised British, occupiers of his homeland.

But now he had made the mistake of trying to run, and five soldiers from the provost marshal's unit, on the lookout for him, had grabbed him from where he had been hiding behind the barn on a farm up in the foothills. The court-martial had been assembled all too quickly and, as with all drumhead justice, the sentence was handed down in a brutally short time: He was to be flogged, thirty lashes with the cat— but only after being seared with a branding iron, the mark of desertion forever to scar his face.

He pleaded with the court; he pleaded with his guards. He cried, he screamed, he struggled. But the soldiers held him down, and Doctor Minor took the hot iron from a basket of glowing coals that had been hastily borrowed from the brigade farrier. He hesitated for a moment—a hesitation that betrayed his own reluctance—for was this, he wondered briefly, truly permitted under the terms of his Hippocratic oath? The officers grunted for him to continue—and he pressed the glowing metal onto the Irishman's cheek. The flesh sizzled, the blood bubbled and steamed; the prisoner screamed and screamed.

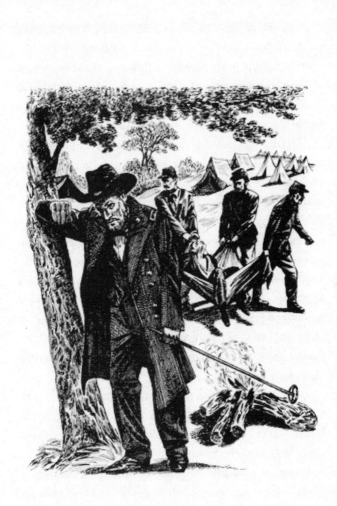

And then it was over. The wretch was led away, holding to his injured cheek the alcohol-soaked rag that Minor had given him. Perhaps the wound would become infected, would fill with the "laudable pus" that other doctors said hinted at cure. Perhaps it would fester and crust with sores. Perhaps it would blister and burst and bleed for weeks. He didn't know.

All that he was sure of was that the brand would be with him for the rest of his life. While in the United States it would mark him as a coward, as shaming a punishment as the court had decreed, back home in Ireland it would mark him as something else altogether: It would mark him as a man who had gone to America to train with the army, and who was now back in Ireland, bent on fighting against the British authorities. He could clearly be identified, from now on, as a member of one of the Irish nationalist rebel groups. Every soldier and policeman in England and Ireland would recognize that, and would either lock him up to keep him off the streets, or would harass and harry him for every moment of his waking life.

His future as an Irish revolutionary was, in other words, over. He cared little for his ruined social standing in the United States; but for his future and now very vulnerable position in Ireland, he had been marked and blighted forever by the fact of one battlefield punishment, and he was bitterly angry. He realized that as an Irish patriot and revolutionary he was useless, unemployable, worthless in all regards.

And in his anger he most probably felt, justly or not, that his ever-more-intense wrath should be directed against the man who had so betrayed his calling as a medical man and had instead, and without objection, marked his face so savagely and incurably. He would have decided that he was and should be bitterly and eternally angry at William Chester Minor.

So he would go home, he vowed, just as soon as this war was over; and once home he would, the moment he stepped off the boat on the docks at Cobh or Dun Laoghaire (or Queenstown or Kingstown, the ports for Cork and Dublin), tell all Irish patriots the following: William Chester Minor, American, was an enemy of all good Fenian fighting men, and revenge should be exacted from him, in good time and in due course.

This, at least, is what Doctor Minor almost certainly thought was in the mind of the man he had branded. Yes, it was later said, he had been terrified by his exposure to the battlefield, and "exposure in the field" was suggested by some doctors as the cause of his ills; one story also had it that he had been present at the execution of a man—a Yale classmate, according to some reports, though none included a time or a place—and that he had been severely affected by what he had seen; but most frequently it was said he was fearful that Irishmen would abuse him shamefully, as he put it, and this was because he had been ordered to inflict so cruel a punishment on one of their number in the United States.

It was a story that was put about in court—Mrs. Fisher, his landlady in Tennison Street, Lambeth, had, according to the official court reports in *The Times*, suggested as much. The

story was raised many times over the following decades—
when people remembered that he was still locked up in an
asylum—to account for his illness; and until 1915, when as
an elderly man he gave an interview to a journalist in Washington, D.C., and told quite another story, it remained one of
the leading probable causes for his insanity. "He branded an
Irishman during the American Civil War," they used to say.
"It drove him mad."

A week or so later Minor—suffering no apparent short-term
effects from his experience—was moved from under the red
flag of the advanced field hospital (the red cross symbol was
not to be adopted by the United States until the ratification of
the Geneva Convention in the late 1860s) and sent to where
he had been originally bound, the city of Alexandria.

He arrived there on May 17, and went first to work at
L'Overture Hospital, then reserved largely for black and so-
called "contraband" patients—escaped Southern slaves.
There are records showing that he moved around the Federal
hospital system: He worked at Alexandria General Hospital
and at the Slough Hospital; there is also a letter from his old
military hospital in New Haven, asking that he come back,
since his work had been so good.

Demand like this was unusual, since Minor was labor-
ing still at the lowliest rank of the war's medical personnel,
as an acting assistant surgeon. In the course of the conflict
5,500 men were Federally contracted at this rank, and they
included some devastating incompetents—specialists in botany and homeopathy, drunks who had failed in private prac-

tice, fraudsters who preyed on their patients, men who had never been to medical school at all. Most would vanish from the army once the fighting was over: Few would even dare hope for promotion or a regular commission.

But William Minor did. He seems to have flung himself into his work. Some of his old autopsy reports survive—they display neat handwriting, a confident use of the language, decisive declarations as to the cause of death. Most of the reports are forlorn—a sergeant from the First Michigan Cavalry dying of lung cancer, a common soldier dying of typhoid, another with pneumonia—all too common ailments during the Civil War period, and all treated with the ignorance of the day, with little more than the dual weapons of opium and calomel, painkiller and purgative.

One report is more interesting: It was written in September 1866—two years after the Wilderness battle—and it concerns a recruit, "a stout muscular man" named Martin Kuster, who was struck by lightning while he was on sentry duty, imprudently standing under a poplar tree during a thunderstorm. He was in bad shape. "The left side of his cap open . . . facing of the metal button torn off . . . hair of his left temple singed and burned . . . stocking and right boot torn open . . . a faint yellow and amber colored line extended down his body . . . burns down to his pubis and scrotum."

This report did not come from Virginia, however, nor was it written by an acting assistant surgeon. It came instead from Governor's Island, New York, and it was signed by Minor in his new capacity as an assistant surgeon in the U.S. Army. By the autumn of 1866 he was no longer a contract man, but instead enjoyed the full rank of a commissioned captain. He had done what most of his colleagues had failed to do: By dint of hard work and scholarship, and by using his Connecticut connections to the full, he had made the transition into the upper ranks of regular army officers.

His supporters, in Connecticut and elsewhere, were unaware of any incipient madness: Professor James Dana—a Yale geologist and mineralogist whose classic textbooks are still in use today, worldwide—said that Minor was "one of the half dozen best . . . in the country," and that his appointment as an army surgeon "would be for the good of the Army and the honor of the country." Another professor wrote of him as "a skillful physician, an excellent operator, an efficient scholar"—although, adding what might later be interpreted as a tocsin note, remarked that his moral character was "unexceptional."

Just before his formal examination Minor had signed a form declaring that he did not labor under any "mental or physical infirmity of any kind, which can in any way interfere with the most efficient duties in any climate." His examiners agreed: In February 1866 they granted him his commission, and by mid-summer he was on Governor's Island, dealing with one of the major emergencies of the postwar period: the fourth and last of the East's great cholera epidemics.

It was said that the illness was brought by Irish immigrants who were then pouring in through Ellis Island: Some twelve hundred people died during the summertime scourge, and the hospitals and clinics on Governor's Island were filled with the sick and the isolated. Minor worked tirelessly throughout the months of the plague, and his work was recognized: By the end of the year, though still nominally a lieutenant, he was breveted with the rank of captain as reward for his services.

But at the same time there came disturbing signs in Minor's behavior, of what with hindsight appears to have been an incipient paranoia. He began to carry a gun when he was out of uniform. Quite illegally, he took along his Colt .38 service revolver, with a six-shot spinning magazine that, according to custom, had one of the chambers blocked off with a permanent blank. He carried the weapon, he explained, because one of his fellow officers had been killed by muggers when returning from a bar in Lower Manhattan. He too might be followed by ruffians, he said, who might try to attack him.

He started to become a habitué of the wilder bars and brothels of the Lower East Side and Brooklyn. He embarked on a career of startling promiscuity, sleeping night after night with whores and returning to the Fort Jay's hospital on Governor's Island by rowboat in the early hours of the morning. His colleagues became alarmed: This was totally out of character, it seemed, for so gentle and studious an officer—and particularly so when it became clear that he frequently needed treatment, or such as was available, for a variety of venereal infections.

In 1867—the year his father, Eastman, died, in New Haven—he surprised his colleagues by suddenly announcing his engagement to a young woman who lived in Manhattan. Neither she nor her job has been identified, but the suspicion is that she was a dancer or an entertainer, met on one of his Tenderloin expeditions. The girl's mother, however, was not so impressed with Minor as his Connecticut friends had been. She detected something unsavory about the young captain and insisted that her daughter break the engagement, which she eventually did. In later years Minor refused adamantly to discuss either the affair or his feelings about its forced conclusion. His doctors said, however, that he appeared embittered about the episode.

The army, meanwhile, was dismayed by what seemed the sudden change in its protégé. Within weeks of learning of his extraordinary behavior the Surgeon General's Department decided to remove him from the temptations of New York and send him out of harm's way, into the countryside. He was effectively demoted, in fact, by being ordered to the relative isolation of obscure Fort Barrancas, Florida. The fort, which guards Pensacola Bay, on the Gulf of Mexico, was already becoming obsolete. An elderly masonry structure built to protect the bay and its port from foreign raiders, it now housed only a small detachment of troops, to whom Minor became regimental doctor. For a man so well born, so educated, so full of promise, this was a truly humiliating situation.

He became furiously angry with the army. He clearly missed his debauches; his messmates noticed that he became moody and occasionally very aggressive. In his quieter moments he took up his paintbrushes: Watercolors of the Florida sunsets soothed him, he said. He still was a dab hand, his brother officers said. He was an artistic man, said one in particular. He seemed like someone with a soul.

But he then began to harbor suspicions about his fellow soldiers. He said he thought they were muttering about him, glancing suspiciously at him all the time. One officer in particular troubled Minor, began teasing him, goading him, persecuting him in ways that Minor would never discuss. He challenged the man to a duel and had to be reprimanded by the fort commander. The officer was one of Minor's best friends, said the commander—and both he and the friend later said they were incredulous that they had fallen out so badly, for no obvious reason. Nothing anyone could do to explain—your best friend is not plotting against you, is not scheming, is not wanting to have you hurt—nothing seemed to get through. Minor appeared to have taken a leave of his senses. It was all very puzzling, and to his friends and family, deeply distressing.

It reached a climax during the summer of 1868, when, after reportedly staying too long in the Florida sun, the captain began to complain of severe headaches and terrible vertigo. He was sent with escorting nurses to New York, to report to his old unit and to his old doctor. He was interviewed, examined, prodded, pried into. By September it was perfectly plain to see that he was seriously unwell. For the first time suspicion turns to certainty, with a formal indication that his mind was starting to falter.

A paper signed by a Surgeon Hammond on September 3, 1868, states that Minor appeared to be suffering from *monomania*—a form of insanity that involves a fierce obsession with a single topic. What that topic was Surgeon Hammond does not report, but he does say that in his view, Minor's condition was so serious that he was to be classified as "delusional." Minor was just thirty-four years old: His mind and his life had begun to spiral out of control.

The sick notes then begin to pile up, week after week— "He is in my opinion, unfit for duty and not able to travel," they each declared. By November the doctors were recommending a more drastic step: Minor should in the army's opinion be immediately institutionalized. He should, moreover, be put in the charge of the celebrated Dr. Charles Nichols, the superintendent of the Government Hospital for the Insane in Washington, D.C.

"The monomania," said the examining doctor, in a letter written in suitably magnificent copperplate, "is now decidedly suicidal and homicidal. Doctor Minor has expressed willingness to go to the Asylum, and has said he hoped he would be permitted to go without a guard, which I think he is now fully capable of doing."

Capable, but ashamed. A letter, begging permission on Minor's behalf for him to go to the asylum without people knowing, survives. "He shrinks from what he regards as the stigma of medical treatment in a lunatic asylum. He does not know that I write this. He would be grateful to anyone whose influence would place him under medical treatment in the Asylum without its being generally known."

The letter worked, the influence of the old family, the old school, proved effective. A day later, without a guard and in secret, Doctor Minor took the express train down through Philadelphia, Wilmington, and Baltimore to Union Station, Washington. He took a hansom cab to southeast

Washington, and to the well-tended grounds of the hospital. He passed through the stone gates, to begin what would become a lifelong acquaintance with the insides of lunatic asylums.

The Washington institution, eventually renamed St. Elizabeth's, would become infamous—Ezra Pound would be detained there, as would John Hinckley, the attempted assassin of President Reagan. For the balance of the nineteenth century, however, the institution would be known more anonymously, as the only government-run site in the country in which soldiers and sailors who had gone certifiably mad could be detained, rehabilitated, locked away. William Minor was to remain there for the next eighteen months. He was a trusted inmate, however: The superintendent allowed him free run of the grounds, then let him go unescorted into the nearby countryside—a century and a half ago Washington was a very different place—fields where now there are slums. He walked into town; he passed by the White House; he visited the pay office each month and drew his salary in cash.

But he remained beset by delusional fears. A team of army doctors visited him the following September. "Our observations lead us to form a very unfavorable opinion as to Dr. Minor's condition," they told the surgeon general. "A very long time may elapse before he can possibly be restored to health." Another doctor concurred: "The disturbance of the cerebral functions is ever more marked."

The following April his commanders reached an unoptimistic decision: Minor was never likely to be cured, they said, and should be formally placed on the Army Retired List. A hearing was held in the Army Building at the corner of Houston and Greene Streets, in what is now New York's fashionable, upscale SoHo area, to formalize the soldier's retirement and to make sure it was justified by circumstance.

It was a protracted, sad affair. A brigadier, two colonels, a major, and a surgeon captain sat on the board, and they listened silently as doctor after doctor gave evidence about this once-so-promising young man's decline. Perhaps the mental condition from which he was suffering had been caused by exposure to the sun in Florida, said one; perhaps it had merely been aggravated by it, said another; perhaps it was all due to the man's exposure to war, a consequence of the horrors that he had witnessed.

No matter precisely how the madness was precipitated, the board eventually reached what was the only proper conclusion on how to deal with it, administratively. In the official view of the army, Brevet Capt. Asst. William C. Minor was now wholly "incapacitated by causes arising in the line of duty"—the crucial phrase of the ruling—and he should be retired with immediate effect.

He was, in other words, one of the walking wounded. He had served his country, he had been ruined by doing so, and his country owed him a debt. If the beguiling eroticisms of Ceylon, his tragic family circumstances, his obsessive cravings for whores, his *nostalgie de la boue*—if any or all of these factors had ever played a part in his steady mental decline, then so be it. The line of duty had done for him. The U.S. Army would now look after him. He was a ward of Uncle Sam. He could be designated by the honorific phrase after his name, "US Army, Ret'd." His pay and pension would remain—and in fact they did so for the rest of his life.

In February 1871 a friend in New York wrote to report that Minor had been released from the asylum, and was on his way to Manhattan, to stay with a medical friend on West Twentieth Street. A few weeks later he was said to have gone home to New Haven, to spend the summer with his brother Alfred, to see his old friends at Yale, and to busy himself in his late father's emporium—Minor & Co., Dealers in China, Glass and Crockery—which Alfred and his older brother George ran at 261 Chapel Street. The summer and autumn days of 1871 were among the last free and tranquil American days that Doctor Minor was ever to enjoy.

In October, with the red-and-gold leaves of the New England trees already beginning to fall, William Minor boarded a steamer in Boston, with a single ticket to the Port of London. He planned to spend a year or so in Europe, he told his friends. He would rest, read, paint. Perhaps he would visit a spa or two, he would see Paris, Rome, and Venice, he would refresh and reinvigorate what he well knew was a troubled mind. One of his friends at Yale had written a letter of introduction to Mr. Ruskin; he would doubtless be able to charm the artistic demimonde of the British capital. He was, after all—and how many times had he heard the phrase at the army hearings—"a gentleman of Christian refinement, taste and learning." He would take London by storm. He would recover. He would return to the United States a new man.

He stepped off the boat on a foggy morning in early November. He offered his identification as an officer in the U.S. Army to the officials in the customs shed, and took a landau to Radley's Hotel, near Victoria Station. He had money with him. He had his books, his easel, his watercolors, his brushes. And he also had, secure in its japanned box, his gun.

4

Gathering
Earth's Daughters

Sesquipedalian (se:skwipĭdēⁱ·liǎn), *a. and sb.* [f. L. *sesquipedālis*: see SESQUIPEDAL and -IAN.]

A. *adj.* **1.** Of words and expressions (after Horace's *sesquipedalia verba* 'words a foot and a half long', A. P. 97): Of many syllables.

B. *sb.* **1.** A person or thing that is a foot and a half in height or length.

1615 *Curry-Combe for Coxe-Combe* iii. 113 He thought fit by his variety, to make you knowne for a viperous Sesquipedalian in euery coast. **1656** Blount *Glossogr*

2. A sesquipedalian word.

1830 *Fraser's Mag.* I. 350 What an amazing power in writing down hard names and sesquipedalians does not the following passage manifest! **1894** *Nat. Observer* 6 Jan. 194/2 His sesquipedalians recall the utterances of another Doctor.

Hence **Se:squipeda·lianism**, style characterized by the use of long words; lengthiness

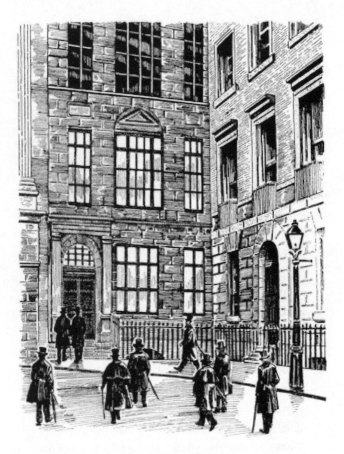

✦

It was also on a foggy day in November, nearly a quarter of a century earlier, that the central events on the other side of this curious conjunction got properly under way. But while Doctor Minor arrived in London on a wintry November morning and took himself to an unfashionable lodging house in Victoria, this very different set of events took place early on a wintry November evening, and in an exceedingly select quarter of Mayfair.

The date was November 5, Guy Fawkes Day, 1857, the time was shortly after six, and the place a narrow terraced house at the northwest corner of one of London's most fashionable and aristocratic oases, St. James's Square. On all sides were the grand townhouses and private clubs of the extraordinary number of bishops and peers and members of Parliament who lived there. The finest shops in town were just a stone's throw away, as well as the prettiest churches, the most splendid offices, the oldest and most haughty of foreign embassies. The corner building on St. James's Square housed an institution that was central to the intellectual lives of the great men who lived nearby (a role it still plays today, though happily in a somewhat more democratic world). It provided accommodation for what its admirers regarded then as they still do today the finest private collection of publicly accessible books in the world, the London Library.

The library had moved there twelve years before, from cramped quarters on Pall Mall. The new building was tall and capacious, and although today it is filled to bursting with many more than a million books, back in 1857 it had only a few thousand volumes and plenty of space to spare. So its committee decided early on to raise extra money by renting out rooms, though only, it was decreed, to societies whose adherents were likely to share the same lofty aims of scholarship as did the library itself, and whose members would be able to mingle happily with the aristocratic and often staggeringly snobbish gentlemen who made up the library's own membership rolls.

Two groups were chosen: The Statistical Society was one, the Philological Society the other. It was at a fortnightly meeting of the latter, held in an upstairs room on that chilly Thursday evening, that words were spoken that were to set in train a most remarkable series of events.

The speaker was the dean of Westminster, a formidable cleric by the name of Richard Chenevix Trench. Perhaps more than any other man alive, Doctor Trench personified the sweepingly noble ambitions of the Philological Society. He firmly believed, as did most of its two hundred members, that some kind of divine ordination lay behind what seemed then the ceaseless dissemination of the English language around the planet.

God—who in that part of London society was of course firmly held to be an Englishman—naturally approved the spread of the language as an essential imperial device; but he also encouraged its undisputed corollary, which was the worldwide growth of Christianity. The equation was really very simple, a formula for undoubted global good: The more English there was in the world, the more God-fearing its peoples would be. (And for a Protestant cleric there was a useful subtext: If English did manage eventually to outstrip the linguistic influences of the Roman Church, then its reach might even help bring the two churches back into some kind of ecumenical—if Anglican-dominated—harmony.)

So, even though the society's stated role was academic, its informal purpose, under the direction of divines like Doctor Trench, was much more robustly chauvinist. True, earnestly classical philological discussions—of obscure topics like "Sound-Shifts in the Papuan and Negrito Dialects," or "The Role of the Explosive Fricative in High German"—did lend the society scholarly heft, which was all very well. But the principal purpose of the group was in fact improving the understanding of what all members regarded as the properly dominant language of the world, and that was their own.

Sixty members were assembled at six o'clock on that November evening. Darkness had fallen on London soon after half past five. The gas lamps fizzed and sputtered, and on the corners of Piccadilly and Jermyn Street small boys were still collecting last-minute pennies for fireworks, their ragged models of old Guy Fawkes—soon to be burned on bonfires—propped up before them. Already in the distance the whistles and crashes and hisses of exploding rockets and Roman candles could be heard, as early parties got under way.

Like the fire-frightened housemaids who hurried back down to the servants' entrances of the great houses nearby, the old philologists, cloaked against the chill, scuttled through the gloom. They were men who had long since outgrown such energetic diversions. They were eager to get away from the sound of explosions and the excitement of celebration, and repair to the calm of scholarly discourse.

Moreover, the topic for their evening's entertainment looked promising, and not in the least taxing. Doctor Trench was to discuss, in a two-part lecture that had been billed as of considerable importance, the subject of dictionaries. The title of his talk suggested a bold agenda: He would tell his audience that those few dictionaries that then existed suffered from a number of serious shortcomings—grave deficiencies from which both the language and—by implication—the empire and its church might well eventually come to suffer. For those Victorians who accepted the sturdy precepts of the Philological Society, this was just the kind of talk they liked to hear.

The "English dictionary," in the sense that we commonly use the phrase today—as an alphabetically arranged list of English words, together with an explanation of their meanings—is a relatively new invention. Four hundred years ago there was no such convenience available on any English bookshelf.

There was none available, for instance, when William Shakespeare was writing his plays. Whenever he came to use an unusual word, or to set a word in what seemed an unusual context—and his plays are extraordinarily rich with examples—he had almost no way of checking the propriety of what he was about to do. He was not able to reach into his bookshelves and select any one volume to help: He would not be able to find any book that might tell him if the word he had chosen was properly spelled, whether he had selected it correctly, or had used it in the right way in the proper place.

Shakespeare was not even able to perform a function that we consider today as perfectly normal and ordinary a function as reading itself. He could not, as the saying goes, "look something up." Indeed the very phrase—when it is used in the sense of "searching for something in a dictionary or encyclopedia or other book of reference"—simply did not exist. It does not appear in the English language, in fact, until as late as 1692, when an Oxford historian named Anthony Wood used it.

Since there was no such phrase until the late seventeenth century, it follows that there was essentially no such concept either, certainly not at the time when Shakespeare was writing—a time when writers were writing furiously, and thinkers thinking as they rarely had before. Despite all the intellectual activity of the time there was in print no guide to the tongue, no linguistic *vade mecum*, no single book that Shakespeare or Martin Frobisher, Francis Drake, Walter Raleigh, Francis Bacon, Edmund Spenser, Christopher Marlowe, Thomas Nash, John Donne, Ben Jonson, Izaak Walton, or any of their other learned contemporaries could consult.

Consider, for instance, Shakespeare's writing of *Twelfth Night*, which he completed sometime at the very beginning of the seventeenth century. Consider the moment, probably in the summer of 1601, when he has reached the writing of the scene in the third act in which Sebastian and Antonio, the shipwrecked sailor and his rescuer, have just arrived in port and are wondering where they might stay the night.

Sebastian considers the question for a moment, and then, in the manner of someone who has read and well remembered his *Good Hotel Guide* of the day, declares quite simply: "In the south suburbs at the Elephant/Is best to lodge."

Now what, exactly, did William Shakespeare know about elephants? Moreover, what did he know of Elephants as hotels? The name was one that was given to a number of lodging houses in various cities dotted around Europe. This particular Elephant, given that this was *Twelfth Night*, happened to be in Illyria; but there were many others, two of them at least in London. But however many there were— just why was this the case? Why name an inn after such a beast? And what was such a beast anyway? All of these are questions that, one would think, a writer should at least have been *able* to answer.

Yet they were not. If Shakespeare did not happen to know very much about elephants, which was likely, and if he were unaware of this curious habit of naming hotels after them— just where could he go to look the question up? And more—if he wasn't precisely sure that he was giving his Sebastian the proper reference for his lines—for was the inn really likely to be named after an elephant, or was it perhaps named after another animal, a camel or a rhino, or a gnu?—where could he look to make quite sure? Where in fact would a playwright of Shakespeare's time look *any* word up?

One might think he would want to look things up all the time. "Am not I consanguineous?" he writes in the same play. A few lines on he talks of "thy doublet of changeable taffeta." He then declares: "Now is the woodcock near the gin."

Shakespeare's vocabulary was evidently prodigious: But how could he be certain that in all the cases where he employed unfamiliar words, he was grammatically and factually right? What prevented him, to nudge him forward by a couple of centuries, from becoming an occasional Mr. Malaprop?

The questions are worth posing simply to illustrate what we would now think of as the profound inconvenience of his not once being able to refer to a dictionary. At the time he was writing there were atlases aplenty, there were prayer books, missals, histories, biographies, romances, and books of science and art. Shakespeare is thought to have drawn many of his classical allusions from a specialized *Thesaurus* that had been compiled by a man named Thomas Cooper—its many errors are replicated far too exactly in the plays for it to be coincidence—and he is thought also to have drawn from Thomas Wilson's *Arte of Rhetorique*. But that was all; there were no other literary, linguistic, and lexical conveniences available.

In the sixteenth century in England, dictionaries such as we would recognize today simply did not exist. If the language that so inspired Shakespeare had limits, if its words had definable origins, spellings, pronunciations, *meanings*— then no single book existed that established them, defined them, and set them down. It is perhaps difficult to imagine so creative a mind working without a single work of lexicographical reference beside him, other than Mr. Cooper's crib (which Mrs. Cooper once threw into the fire, prompting the great man to begin all over again) and Mr. Wilson's little manual, but that was the condition under which his particular genius was compelled to flourish. The English language was spoken and written—but at the time of Shakespeare it was not defined, not *fixed*. It was like the air—it was taken for granted, the medium that enveloped and defined all Britons. But as to exactly what it was, what its components were— who knew?

That is not to say there were no dictionaries at all. There had been a collection of Latin words published as a *Dictionarius* as early as 1225, and a little more than a century later another, also Latin-only, as a helpmeet for students of Saint Jerome's difficult translation of the Scriptures known as the Vulgate. In 1538 the first of a series of Latin-English dictionaries appeared in London—Thomas Elyot's alphabetically arranged list, which happened to be the first book to employ the English word *dictionary* in its title. Twenty years later a man named Withals put out *A Shorte Dictionarie for Yonge Beginners* in both languages, but with the words arranged not alphabetically but by subject, such as "the names of Byrdes, Byrdes of the Water, Byrdes about the house, as cockes, hennes, etc., of Bees, Flies, and others."

But what was still lacking was a proper English dictionary, a full statement of the extent of the English tongue. With one single exception, of which Shakespeare probably did not know when he died in 1616, this need remained stubbornly unfulfilled. Others were to remark on the apparent lack as well. In the very same year as Shakespeare's death, his friend John Webster wrote his *The Duchess of Malfi*, incorporating a scene in which the duchess's brother Ferdinand imagines that he is turning into a wolf, "a pestilent disease they call licanthropia." "What is that?" cries one of the cast. "I need a dictionary to't!"

But in fact someone, a Rutland schoolmaster named Robert Cawdrey, who later moved to teach in Coventry, had evidently been listening to this drumbeat of demand. He read and took copious notes from all the reference books of the day and eventually produced his first halfhearted attempt at what was wanted by publishing such a list in 1604 (the year Shakespeare probably wrote *Measure for Measure*).

It was a small octavo book of 120 pages, which Cawdrey titled *A Table Alphabeticall . . . of hard unusual English Words*. It had about 2,500 word entries. He had compiled it, he said, "for the benefit & help of Ladies, gentlewomen or any other unskilful persons, Whereby they may more easilie and better understand many hard English wordes, which they shall heare or read in the Scriptures, Sermons or elsewhere, and also be made able to use the same aptly themselves." It had many shortcomings; but it was without doubt the very first true monolingual English dictionary, and its publication remains a pivotal moment in the history of English lexicography.

For the next century and a half there was a great flurry of commercial activity in the field, and dictionary after dictionary thundered off the presses, each one larger than the next, each boasting of superior value in the educating of the uneducated (among whom were counted the women of the day, most of whom enjoyed little schooling, compared to the men).

Throughout the seventeenth century these books tended to concentrate, as Cawdrey's first offering had, on what were called "hard words"—words that were not in common, everyday use, or else words that had been invented specifically to impress others, the so-called "inkhorn terms" with which sixteenth- and seventeenth-century books seem well larded. Thomas Wilson, whose *Arte of Rhetorique* had helped Shakespeare, published examples of the high-flown style, such as that from a clergyman in Lincolnshire writing to a government official, begging a promotion:

> There is a Sacerdotall dignitie in my native Countrey contiguate to me, where I now contemplate: which your worshipfull benignitie could sone impenetrate for mee, if it would like you to extend your sedules, and collaude me in them to the right honourable lord Chaunceller, or rather Archgrammacian of Englande.

The fact that the volumes concentrated on only the small section of the national vocabulary that encompassed such nonsense might seem today to render them bizarrely incomplete, but back then their editorial selection was regarded as a virtue. Speaking and writing thus was the highest ambition of the English smart set. "We present for you," trumpeted the editor of one such volume to would-be members, "the choicest words."

So, fantastic linguistic creations like *abequitate*, *bulbulcitate*, and *sullevation* appeared in these books alongside *archgrammacian* and *contiguate*, with lengthy definitions; there were words like *necessitude*, *commotrix*, and *parentate*—all of which are now listed, if listed at all, as "obsolete" or "rare" or both. Pretentious and flowery inventions adorned the language—perhaps not all that surprising, considering the flowery fashion of the times, with its perukes and powdered periwigs; its rebatos and doublets; its ruffs, ribbons; and scarlet velvet Rhinegraves. So words like *adminiculation, cautionate, deruncinate,* and *attemptate* are placed in the vocabulary too, each duly cataloged in the tiny leather books of the day; yet they were words meant only for the loftiest ears, and were unlikely to impress Cawdrey's intended audience of ladies, gentlewomen, and "unskillful persons."

The definitions offered by these books were generally unsatisfactory too. Some offered mere one-word or barely illuminating synonyms—*magnitude*: "greatness," or *ruminate*: "to chew over again, to studie earnestly upon." Sometimes the definitions were simply amusing: Henry Cockeram's *The English Dictionarie* of 1623 defines *commotrix* as "A Maid that makes ready and unready her Mistress," while *parentate* is "To celebrate one's parents' funerals." Or else the creators of these hardword books put forward explanations that were complex beyond endurance, as in a book called *Glossographia* by Thomas Blount, which offers as its definition of *shrew*: "a kind of Field-Mouse, which if he goes over a beasts back, will make him lame in the Chine; and if he bite, the beast swells to the heart, and dyes. . . . From hence came our English phrase, I beshrew thee, when we wish ill; and we call a curst woman a Shrew."

Yet in all of this lexicographical sound and fury—seven major dictionaries had been produced in seventeenth-century

England, the last having no fewer than thirty-eight thousand headwords—two matters were being ignored.

The first was the need for a good dictionary to encompass the language *in its entirety*, the easy and popular words as well as the hard and obscure, the vocabulary of the common man as well as that of the learned house, the aristocrat, and the rarefied school. Everything should be included: The mite of a two-letter preposition should have no less standing in an ideal word list than the majesty of a piece of polysyllabic sesquipedalianism.

The second matter that dictionary makers were ignoring was the coming recognition elsewhere that, with Britain and its influence now beginning to flourish in the world—with daring sailors like Drake and Raleigh and Frobisher skimming the seas; with European rivals bending before the might of British power; and with new colonies securely founded in the Americas and India, which spread the English language and English concepts far beyond the shores of England—English was trembling on the verge of becoming a global language. It was starting to be an important vehicle for the conduct of international commerce, arms, and law. It was displacing French, Spanish, and Italian and the courtly languages of foreigners; it needed to be far better known, far better able to be properly learned. An inventory needed to be made of what was spoken, what was written, and what was read.

The Italians, the French, and the Germans were already well advanced in securing their own linguistic heritage, and had gone so far as to ordain institutions to maintain their languages in fine fettle. In Florence the Accademia della Crusca had been founded in 1582, dedicated to maintaining "Italian" culture, even though it would be three centuries before there was a political entity called Italy. But a dictionary of Italian was produced by the Accademia in 1612: The linguistic culture was alive, if not the country. In Paris, Richelieu had established the Académie Française in 1634. The Forty Immortals—rendered in perhaps more sinister fashion as simply "the Forty"—have presided over the integrity of the tongue with magnificent inscrutability until this day.

But the British had taken no such approach. It was in the eighteenth century that the impression grew that the nation needed to know in more detail what its language was, and what it meant. The English at the close of the seventeenth century, it was said, were "uncomfortably aware of their backwardness in the study of their own tongue." From then on the air was full of schemes for bettering the English language, for giving it greater prestige both at home and abroad.

Dictionaries improved, and very markedly so, during the first half of the new century. The most notable of them, a book that did indeed expand its emphasis from mere hard words to a broad swathe of the entire English vocabulary, was edited by a Stepney boarding-school owner named Nathaniel Bailey. Very little is known about him, other than his membership in the Seventh-Day Baptist Church. But the breadth of his scholarship, the scope of his interest, is amply indicated by the title page of his first edition (there were to be twenty-five between 1721 and 1782, all bestsellers). The page also hints at the quite formidable task that lay ahead of any drudge who might be planning to create a truly comprehensive English lexicon. Bailey's work was entitled:

> A Universal Etymological Dictionary, Comprehending The Derivations of the Generality of Words in the English tongue, either Antient or Modern, from the Antient British, Saxon, Danish, Norman and Modern French, Teutonic, Dutch, Spanish, Italian, Latin, Greek and Hebrew Languages, each in their proper Characters. And Also A brief and clear Explication of all difficult Words . . . and Terms of Art relating to Botany, Anatomy, Physick . . . Together with A Large Collection and Explication of Words and Phrases us'd in our Antient Statutes, Charters, Writs, Old Records and Processes at Law; and the Etymology and Interpretation of the Proper Names of Men, Woman and Remarkable Places in Great Britain; also the Dialects of our Different Counties. Containing many Thousand Words more than . . . any English Dictionary before extant. To which is Added a Collection of our most Common Proverbs, with their Explication and Illustration. The whole work compil'd and Methodically digested, as well as for the Entertainment of the Curious as the Information of the Ignorant, and for the Benefit of young Students, Artificers, Tradesmen and Foreigners. . .

Good the volumes and the effort may have been, but still not quite good enough. Nathaniel Bailey and those who tried to copy him in the first half of the eighteenth century labored mightily at their task, though the task of corralling the entire language became ever larger the more it was considered. Yet still no one seemed intellectually capable, or brave, or dedicated enough, or simply possessed of enough time, to make a truly full record of the entire English language. And that, though no one seemed able even to say so, was what was really wanted. An end to timidity, to pussyfooting—the replacement of the philologically tentative by the lexicographically decisive.

And then came the man whom Tobias Smollett called "Literature's Great Cham"—one of the most eminent literary figures of all time—Samuel Johnson. He decided to take up the challenge before which so many others had flinched. And even with the critical judgment of the more than two centuries since, it can fairly be said that what he created was an unparalleled triumph. Johnson's *A Dictionary of the English Language* was, and has remained ever since, a portrait of the language of the day in all its majesty, beauty, and marvelous confusion.

Few are the books that can offer so much pleasure to look at, to touch, to skim, to read.

They can still be found today, often cased in boxes of brown morocco. They are hugely heavy, built for the lectern rather than the hand. They are bound in rich brown leather, the paper is thick and creamy, the print impressed deep into the weave. Few who read the volumes today can fail to be charmed by the quaint elegance of the definitions, of which Johnson was a master. Take for example the word for which Shakespeare might have hunted, *elephant*. It was, Johnson declared:

The largest of all quadrupeds, of whose sagacity, faithfulness, prudence and even understanding,
many surprising relations are given. This animal is
not carnivorous, but feeds on hay, herbs and all sorts
of pulse; and it is said to be extremely long lifed. It
is naturally very gentle; but when enraged, no creature is more terrible. He is supplied with a trunk, or
long hollow cartilage, like a large trumpet, which
hangs between his teeth, and serves him for hands:
by one blow with his trunk he will kill a camel or a
horse, and will raise of prodigious weight with it. His
teeth are the ivory so well known in Europe, some of
which have been seen as large as a man's thigh, and a
fathom in length. Wild elephants are taken with the
help of a female ready for the male: she is confined to
a narrow place, round which pits are dug; and these
being covered with a little earth scattered over hur-
dles, the male elephant easily falls into the snare. In
copulation the female receives the male lying upon
her back; and such is his pudicity, that he never covers the female so long as anyone appears in sight.

Yet Johnson's dictionary represents more, far more, than
mere quaintness and charm. Its publication represented a
pivotal moment in the history of the English language; the
only more significant moment was to commence almost exactly a century later.

Samuel Johnson had been thinking about and planning the structure of his dictionary for many years. He had

been doing so in part to create a reputation for himself. He was a schoolteacher turned scribbler, known only in limited metropolitan circles as the parliamentary sketch writer for the *Gentleman's Magazine*. He was eager to have himself better regarded. But he began the process also in response to calls from the giants—demands that something needed to be done.

Theirs was a near-universal complaint. Joseph Addison, Alexander Pope, Daniel Defoe, John Dryden, Jonathan Swift, the leading lights of English literature, had each spoken out, calling for the need to fix the language. By that—*fixing* has been a term of lexicographical jargon ever since—they meant establishing the limits of the language, creating an inventory of its word stock, forging its cosmology, deciding exactly what the language was. Their considered view of the nature of English was splendidly autocratic: The tongue, they insisted, had by the turn of the seventeenth century become sufficiently refined and pure that it could only remain static or else thenceforward deteriorate.

By and large they agreed with the beliefs of the Forty Immortals across the Channel (though they would have been loath to admit it): A national standard language needed to be defined, measured, laid down, chased in silver, and carved in stone. Alterations to it then could be permitted or not, according to the mood of the great and the good, a home-grown Forty, a national language authority.

Swift was the fiercest advocate of all. He once wrote to the earl of Oxford to express his outrage that words like *bamboozle, uppish,* and—of all things—*couldn't* were appearing in print. He wanted the establishment of strict rules banning such words as offensive to good sense. In future he wanted all spellings fixed—a firm orthography, the correctness of writing. He wanted the pronunciations laid down—an equally firm orthoepy, the correctness of speech. Rules, rules, rules: They were essential, declared Gulliver's creator.

The language should be accorded just the same dignity and respect as those other standards that science was then also defining. What is blue or yellow? physicists were then wondering. How hot is boiling water? How long is a yard? How to define what musicians knew as middle C? What, indeed, of the precise measurement of longitude, so vital to seamen? Enormous efforts were being made in this particular field at just the same time as the debate over the national language: A Board of Longitude had been set up by the government, funds were being disbursed, and prizes offered just so that a clock could be invented that would go to sea on a ship and be only almost imperceptibly inaccurate. Longitude was vitally important: So great a trading nation as Britain needed to have its ships' masters know exactly where they were.

And so the thinking of great literary men went—if longitude was important, if the defining of color, length, mass, and sound was vital—why was the same import not given to the national tongue? As one pamphleteer wailed, appropriately: "We have neither Grammar nor Dictionary, neither Chart nor Compass, to guide us through the wide sea of Words."

No dictionary had proved adequate so far, said Swift and his friends, but given the heights of perfection that the language had already achieved, one was now needed, and a dedicated genius must be found and applied to the task of making one. It would accomplish two desirable deeds: the fixing of the language and the maintenance of its purity.

Samuel Johnson could not have disagreed more. At least he wanted to have no truck with ordering the language to remain pure. He might have liked it to, but he knew it couldn't be done. As to whether he thought it possible or desirable to fix it, theses have tumbled by the score from academic presses in recent years, arguing variously that Johnson did want to or that he did not. The consensus now is that he originally planned to make a fix on the tongue, but when he was halfway through his six-year task, he came to realize that it was both impossible and undesirable.

One of his predecessors, Benjamin Martin, explained why: "No language as depending on arbitrary use and custom can ever be permanently the same, but will always be in a mutable and fluctuating state; and what is deem'd polite and elegant in one age, may be accounted uncouth and barbarous in another." This dictum, which appeared in the preface to still another half-baked attempt at a proper dictionary just a year before Johnson brought out his own, might as well have guided the Great Cham through his entire construction.

For all the heady talk among London's intelligentsia, it was actually the free market that prompted Johnson to begin. In 1746 a group of five London booksellers (the famous Messrs. Longman among them) were seized with the idea that a brand-new dictionary would sell like hotcakes: They approached their favorite parliamentary writer, whom they knew to be both eager and broke, and made him an offer he could scarcely refuse: fifteen hundred guineas, half of it up front. Johnson agreed readily, with the sole caveat that he would seek as patron the man who was currently the arbiter of all that was good and worthwhile in literary England, Philip Dormer Stanhope, the fourth earl of Chesterfield.

Lord Chesterfield was one of the most remarkable figures in the land: an ambassador, a lord lieutenant of Ireland, a friend of Pope, Swift, Voltaire, and John Gay. It was Chesterfield who had forced England to adopt the Gregorian calendar, and it was Chesterfield whose letters to his bastard son Philip, advising him on his behavior, became, when published, an indispensable *vade mecum* of good manners. His imprimatur on the dictionary would be valuable, his patronage of the project invaluable.

That he promised the imprimatur but declined the patronage (except for handing Johnson a draft for a measly ten pounds) but then went on to claim a part in Johnson's subsequent triumph became a source of well-publicized hard feelings. Lord Chesterfield, Johnson was to say later, taught "the morals of a whore and the manners of a dancing-master." Chesterfield had the elephantine hide of a true aristocrat, and brushed off the criticisms as good natured, which they were not.

His early advocacy of the dictionary, plus the seven hundred and fifty guineas that the booksellers had placed in Johnson's hand, nonetheless set the thirty-seven-year-old editor to work. He took rooms off Fleet Street, hired six serving men (five of them Scotsmen, which would come as some comfort to James Murray, who was from Hawick) as amanuenses, and settled down to the six years of unremitting drudgery that were to prove necessary. He had decided, as Murray was to decide a century later, that the best way—indeed the only way—to compile a full dictionary was to read: to go through all literature and list the words that appeared on hundreds of thousands of pages.

It is an axiom that you have three overlapping choices in making a word list. You may record words that are heard. You may copy the words from other existing dictionaries. Or you may read, after which, in the most painstaking way, you record all the words you have read, sort them, and make them into a list.

Johnson dismissed the first idea as far too cumbersome to be useful; he naturally agreed to the second—all lexicographers use earlier dictionaries as a starting point, to make sure they miss nothing; and, most significantly, he decided on the primary importance of the third choice, reading. Hence the taking of the rooms off Fleet Street, hence the buying or borrowing of books by the ton and the yard and the sack, and hence the hiring of the six men. The team of seven had been created to browse and graze through all existing writings, and to make a catalog of all that was swept into the team's collective maw.

It was swiftly realized that it would be impossible to look through everything, and so Johnson imposed limits. The language, he decided, had probably reached its peak with the writings of Shakespeare, Bacon, and Edmund Spenser, and so there was probably precious little need to go look further back than their lifetimes. He ruled, therefore, that the works of Sir Philip

Sidney, who was only thirty-two when he died in 1586, would usefully mark the starting point for his search; and the last books published by newly dead authors would mark the end.

His dictionary would thus be the result of a concerted trawl through just a century and a half of writing, with the odd piece of Chaucer thrown in for good measure. So Johnson took down these books and read, then underlined and circled words he wanted, and annotated the pages he had chosen; he then demanded that his men copy onto slips of paper the full sentences that displayed his chosen words; and these he then filed, to use when necessary, to illustrate the point he was making, the meaning of a word that he was trying to show.

And it was all those quoted meanings, a demonstration of the multiplicity of subtle shadings of sense that can be encompassed by the simple arrangement of a group of letters, that prove the great triumph of Johnson's dictionary. For while we might laugh at the quaint charm of his definition of *elephant*, or of *oats* ("a grain which in England is generally given to horses, but in Scotland supports the people"), or *lexicographer* ("a writer of dictionaries; a harmless drudge, that busies himself in tracing the original, and detailing the signification of words"), we can only be staggered by his dealing with, say, the verb *take*. Johnson listed, with supportive quotations, no fewer than 113 senses of this particular verb's transitive form and 21 of the intransitive. "To seize, grasp or capture; to catch with a hook; to catch someone in an error; to win popular favor; to be effective; to claim to do something; to assume the right . . . to mount a horse, to flee, to perform what one does in removing one's clothing. . . ."

The list is almost endless: It was a mark of Samuel Johnson's genius that, armed with references from 150 years of English writings, he was able, and essentially single-handedly, to find and note almost every use of every word of the day. Not simply *take*; but other common coin like *set* and *do* and *go* and hundreds upon hundreds of others. Small wonder that once his project was well under way, and the trifling business of his creditors' needs arose, he once barred the door to the milkman with his bed, crying from behind the door, "Depend on it, I will defend this little citadel to the utmost!"

He finished amassing his list of the English word stock in 1750. He spent the next four years editing the citations and choosing the 118,000 illustrative quotations (sometimes by committing the heresy of changing quotes he didn't like). Finally he completed the definitions of what were to become the 43,500 chosen headwords. He wrote some of these definitions from scratch, or else he borrowed substantial passages for others from writers he admired (as with *elephant*, which was partly the work of a man named Calmet).

He did not publish the completed work until 1755, however: He wanted to persuade Oxford University to grant him a degree, believing that if he was able to add it to his name on the title page, it would do Oxford, the book's sales, and himself—and not necessarily in that order—a lot of good. Oxford agreed; and on April 15, 1755, there appeared:

A Dictionary of the English Language, in which the Words are deduced from their Originals and Illustrated in their Different Significations by Exam-

ples from the best Writers to which are prefixed a
History of the Language and an English Grammar,
by Samuel Johnson, A.M., in Two Volumes.

The book, which went into four editions during Johnson's lifetime, was to remain the standard work, an unrivaled
repository of the English language for the next century. It was
an enormous commercial success and was almost universally
praised—particularly by the egregious Lord Chesterfield,
who hinted that he had had rather more to do with the book's
making than he had. This enraged Johnson; not only did he
mutter about whores and dancing masters, but he had up his
sleeve the unkindest cut: Under the definition of *patron* he
had written "a wretch who supports with indolence, and is
paid with flattery." But the noble Lord brushed this aside too,
as Lords are wont to do.

There were some critics. The fact that Johnson allowed
his own personality to invade the pages may today seem
pleasant whimsy, but to some who wanted the book to be
supremely authoritative, it was irritatingly unprofessional.
Many writers sniped at the limited authority of some of those
whom Johnson quoted—a criticism that Johnson himself anticipated in his preface. Some found the definitions patchy—
some trite, some unnecessarily complicated (as with *network*:
"any thing reticulated, or decussated, at equal distances, with
interstices between the intersections"). A century after publication the redoubtable Thomas Babington Macauley was to
damn Johnson as "a wretched etymologist."

But, Macauley aside, many of the critics were probably

just jealous, envious that Johnson had done what none of them could ever do. "Any schoolmaster might have done what Johnson did," wrote one. "His *Dictionary* is merely a glossary to his own barbarous works." But the writer was anonymous and quite probably a disappointed rival. Or else a rabid Whig: Johnson was a noted Tory and wrote with what some thought a distinctive Tory bias. So the book was merely "a vehicle for Jacobite and high-flying tracts," wrote one Whig, doubtless a diehard. One woman even disparaged Johnson for failing to include obscenities. "No, Madam, I hope I have not daubed my fingers," he replied, archly. "I find, however, that you have been looking for them."

Yet the accolades were many. Voltaire proposed that the French model a new dictionary of their own on Johnson's; and the venerable Accademia della Crusca wrote from Florence that Johnson's work will be "a perpetual Monument of Fame to the Author, an Honour to his own Country in particular, and a general Benefit to the republic of Letters throughout all Europe." "In an age of dictionaries of all kinds," wrote a modern consideration, "Johnson's contribution was simply *primus inter pares*." And Robert Burchfield, who edited the four-volume supplement to the *Oxford English Dictionary* in the 1970s, had no doubts: Johnson managed to combine being both a lexicographer and a supremely literate man: "In the whole tradition of the English language and literature the *only* dictionary compiled by a writer of the first rank is that of Dr. Johnson."

Throughout it all, under the rains of slings, arrows, plaudits, and encomiums, Samuel Johnson remained calmly modest. Not unduly so, for he was proud of his work but awed by the magnificence of the language he, with such foolhardiness, had chosen to tackle. The book remained his monument. James Murray was to say in later years that whenever someone used the phrase "the Dictionary," as one might say "the Bible" or "the Prayer Book," he or she referred to the work by Doctor Johnson.

But no, Literature's Great Cham would have said—in fact it was the words that were the truest monument, and even more profoundly, the very entities that those words defined. "I am not yet so lost in lexicography," he says in his famous preface, "as to forget that words are the daughters of earth, and that things are the sons of heaven." His life had been devoted to the gathering in of those daughters, but it was heaven that had ordained their creation.

5

The Big Dictionary Conceived

Elephant (e·lĭ´fănt). Forms: a. 4–6 oli-, olyfaunte, (4 *pl.* olifauns, -fauntz), 4 olyfont, -funt, 5–6 oli-fant(e, 4 olephaunte, 5–6 olyphaunt, 4–7 oli-, olyphant(e. *β*. 4 elifans, 4–5 ele-, elyphaunt(e, 5 elefaunte, 6 eliphant, 5–6 elephante, 6– elephant. [ME. *olifaunt*, a. OF. *olifant*, repr. a popular L. *olifantu-m (whence Pr. *olifan*; cf. MDu. *olfant*, Bret. *olifant*, Welsh *oliffant*, Corn. *oliphans*, which may be all from ME. or OFr.), corrupt form of L. *elephantum, elephantem* (nom. *elephantus, -phas, -phans*), ad. and a. Gr. ἐλέΦας (gen. ἐλέΦαντος). The refashioning of the word after Lat. seems to have taken place earlier in Eng. than in Fr., the Fr. forms with *el-* being cited only from 15th c.

Of the ultimate etymology nothing is really known. As the Gr. word is found (though only in sense 'ivory') in Homer and Hesiod, it seems unlikely that it can be, as some have supposed,

of Indian origin. The resemblance in sound to
Heb. אלף *eleph* 'ox' has given rise to a suggestion
of derivation from some Phœnician or Punic
compound of that word; others have conjectured
that the word may be African. See Yule *Hobson-
Jobson* Suppl., s.v. For the possible relation to this
word of the Teut. and Slavonic name for 'camel',
see OLFEND. The origin of the corrupt Romanic
forms with *ol-* is unknown, but they may be compared with L. *oleum, olīva*, ad. Gr. ἔλαιον, ἐλοία.]
  1. A huge quadruped of the Pachydermate order,
having long curving ivory tusks, and a prehensile
trunk or proboscis. Of several species once distrib-
uted over the world, including Britain, only two
now exist, the Indian and African; the former (the
largest of extant land animals), is often used as a
beast of burden, and in war.

The achievements of the great dictionary makers of England's seventeenth and eighteenth centuries were prodigious indeed. Their learning was unrivaled, their scholarship
sheer genius, their contributions to literary history profound.
All this is undeniable—and yet, cruel though it seems even to
venture to inquire: Who now really remembers their dictionaries, and who today makes use of all that they achieved?

  The question begs an inescapably poignant truth, of
the kind that dims so many other pioneering achievements
in fields that extend beyond and are quite unrelated to this

one. The reality, as seen from today's perspective, is simply: However distinguished the lexicographical works of Thomas Elyot, Robert Cawdrey, Henry Cockeram, and Nathaniel Bailey, and however masterly and pivotal the creation of the Great Cham, Samuel Johnson himself, their achievements seem nowadays to have been only stepping-stones, and their magnificent volumes of work very little more than curios, to be traded, hoarded, and forgotten.

And the reason for this is principally that in 1857, just over a century after the publication of the first edition of Johnson's *Dictionary*, there came a formal proposal for the making of a brand-new work of truly stellar ambition, a lex-icographical project that would be of far, far greater breadth and complexity than anything attempted before.

It had as its goal a quite elegantly simple impertinence: While Johnson had presented a selection of the language— and an enormous selection at that, brilliantly fashioned— this new project would present *all of it*: every word, every nuance, every shading of meaning and spelling and pronun-ciation, every twist of etymology, every possible illustrative citation from every English author.

It was referred to simply as the "big dictionary." When conceived it was a project of almost unimaginable boldness and fool-hardiness, requiring great bravura, risking great hubris. Yet there were men in Victorian England who were properly bold and foolhardy, who were more than up to the implicit risks: This was, after all, a time of great men, great vision, great achievement. Perhaps no time in modern history was more suited to the launching of a project of such grandiosity; which is perhaps why duly, and ponderously, it got under way. Grave problems and seemingly intractable crises threatened more than once to wreck it. Disputations and delays surrounded it. But eventually—by which time many of those great and complicated men who first had the vision were long in their graves—the goal of which Johnson himself might have dreamed—was duly attained.

And while Samuel Johnson and his team had taken six years to create their triumph, those involved in making what was to be, and still is, the ultimate English dictionary took seventy years almost to the day.

The big dictionary's making began with the speech at the London Library, on Guy Fawkes Day, 1857.

Richard Chenevix Trench was officially designated by his contemporary obituarists as "a divine," a term that is rarely used today but that embraced all manner of good and eminent Victorians who pursued all kinds of callings and who wore the cloth while doing so. At the time of his death in 1886, Trench was still regarded more as a divine than anything else—he had had a glittering ecclesiastical career that culminated in his being made dean of Westminster and then archbishop of Dublin. He also was lame because of breaking both his knees: not because of any excess of genuflective piety, however, but because he fell down a gangplank while crossing on the boat to Ireland.

His theme on that lexicographically famous evening was intriguing. Advertised on handbills and in flyers posted around London's West End, it was "On Some Deficiencies in Our English Dictionaries." By today's standards the title seems self-effacing, but given the imperial temper of the time and the firm belief that English was the quintessential imperial language and that any books that dealt with it were important tools for the maintenance of the empire, the title offered an amply understandable hint of the impact that Doctor Trench would be likely to have.

He identified seven principal ways in which the dictionaries then available were to be found wanting—most of them are technical and should not concern us here. But his underlying theme was profoundly simple: It was an essential credo for any future dictionary maker, he said, to realize that a dictionary was simply "an inventory of the language" and decidedly not a guide to proper usage. Its assembler had no business selecting words for inclusion on the basis of whether they were good or bad. Yet all of the craft's earlier practitioners, Samuel Johnson included, had been guilty of doing just that. The lexicographer, Trench pointed out, was "an historian . . . not a critic." It was not within the remit of one dictator—"or Forty" he added, with a cheeky nod at Paris—to determine which words should be used and which should not. A dictionary should be a record of *all* words that enjoy any recognized life span in the standard language.

And the heart of such a dictionary, he went on, should be the history of the life span of each and every word. Some words are ancient and exist still. Others are new and vanish like mayflies. Still others emerge in one lifetime, continue to exist through the next and the next, and look set to endure forever. Others deserve a less optimistic prognosis. Yet all these types of words are valid parts of the English language, no matter that they are old and obsolete or new and with questionable futures. Consider the golden question, said Trench: If someone needs to look up any word, then it should be there—for if not, the work of reference that book purports to be becomes a nonsense, something to which one cannot refer.

Now he was warming to his theme: To chart the life of each word, he continued, to offer its biography, as it were, it is important to know just when the word was born, to have a record of the register of its birth. Not in the sense of when it was first spoken, of course—that, until the advent of the tape-recorder, could never be known—but when it was first written down. Any dictionary that was to be based on the historical principles that, Trench insisted, were the only truly valid ones had to have, for every word, a passage quoted from literature that showed where each word was used first.

And after that, and also for each word, there should be sentences that show the twists and turns of meanings—the way almost every word slips in its silvery, fishlike way, weaving this way and that, adding subtleties of nuance to itself, and then perhaps shedding them as the public mood dictates. "A Dictionary," Trench said, "is an historical monument, the history of a nation contemplated from one point of view, and the wrong ways into which a language has wandered . . . may be nearly as instructive as the right ones."

Johnson's dictionary may have been among the pioneers in presenting quotations (an Italian, for example, claimed that his dictionary had already done so in 1598), but they

were there only to illustrate meaning. The new venture that
Trench seemed now to be proposing would demonstrate not
merely meaning but the history of meaning, the life story of
each word. And that would mean the reading of everything
and the quoting of everything that showed anything of the
history of the words that were to be cited. The task would be
gigantic, monumental, and—according to the conventional
thinking of the times—impossible.

Except that here Trench presented an idea, an idea that—to
those ranks of conservative and frock-coated men who sat silently in the library on that dank and foggy evening—was po-
tentially dangerous and revolutionary. But it was the idea that
in the end made the whole venture possible.

The undertaking of the scheme, he said, was beyond the
ability of any one man. To peruse all of English literature—
and to comb the London and New York newspapers and the
most literate of the magazines and journals—must be instead
"the combined action of many." It would be necessary to recruit a team—moreover, a huge one—probably comprising
hundreds and hundreds of unpaid amateurs, all of them
working as volunteers.

The audience murmured with surprise. Such an idea,
obvious though it may sound today, had never been put forward before. But then, some members said as the meeting was
breaking up, it did have some real merit. It had a rough, rather
democratic appeal. It was an idea consonant with Trench's
underlying thought, that any grand new dictionary ought to
be itself a democratic product, a book that demonstrated the

primacy of individual freedoms, of the notion that one could use words freely, as one liked, without hard and fast rules of lexical conduct.

Any such dictionary certainly should not be an absolutist, autocratic product, such as the French had in mind: The English, who had raised eccentricity and poor organization to a high art, and placed the scatterbrain on a pedestal, loathed such Middle European things as rules, conventions, and dictatorships. They abhorred the idea of diktats—about the language, for Heaven's sake!—emanating from some secretive body of unaccountable immortals. Yes, nodded a number of members of the Philological Society, as they gathered up their astrakhan-collared coats and white silk scarves and top hats that night and strolled out into the yellowish November fog: Dean Trench's notion of calling for volunteers was a good one, a worthy and really rather noble idea.

And it was also, as it happens, an idea that would eventually permit the involvement in the project of one scholarly but troubled lexicographer manqué: Asst. Surgeon (Ret'd.), U.S. Army, Brevet Capt. William Chester Minor.

This, however, was only the idea. It took twenty-two more years of sporadic and sometimes desultory activity before the new dictionary truly got off the ground. The Philological Society had already complicated matters: Six months before Trench's famous speech it had set up an Unregistered Words Committee; had corralled along with Trench the boisterous Frederick Furnivall and Herbert Coleridge, the poet's grandson, to run it; and had planned to devote its corporate efforts to publishing a supplement dictionary, of everything not found in the books that had already been published.

It took many months for the enthusiasm behind that project to abate—though it was given a nudge by the swift realization that so many words were being uncovered in searches that any supplement would be far, far bigger than any book, even Johnson's, that was already available. Once that was behind them, the society formally adopted the idea of a wholly new dictionary: January 7, 1858, when the plan was adopted, is normally reckoned the starting point, at least on paper.

Furnivall then issued a circular calling for volunteer readers. They could select from which period of history they would like to read books—from 1250 to 1526, the year of the New English Testament; from then to 1674, the year when Milton died; or from 1674 to what was then the present day. Each period, it was felt, represented the existence of different trends in the development of the language.

The volunteers' duties were simple enough, if onerous. They would write to the society offering their services in reading certain books; they would be asked to read, and make wordlists of all that they read, and would then be asked to look, super-specifically, for certain words that currently interested the dictionary team. Each volunteer would take a slip of paper, write at its top left-hand side the target word, and below, also on the left, the date of the details that followed: These were, in order, the title of the book or paper, its volume and page number, and then, below that, the full sentence that illustrated the use of the target word. It was a technique that has been undertaken by lexicographers to the present day.

Herbert Coleridge became the first editor of what was to be called *A New English Dictionary on Historical Principles.* He undertook as his first task what may seem prosaic in the extreme: the design of a small stack of oak-board pigeonholes, nine holes wide and six high, which could accommodate the anticipated sixty to one hundred thousand slips of paper that would come in from the volunteers. He estimated that the first volume of the dictionary would be available to the world within two years. "And were it not for the dilatoriness of many contributors," he wrote, clearly in a tetchy mood, "I should not hesitate to name an earlier period."

Everything about these forecasts was magnificently wrong. In the end more than *six million* slips of paper came in from the volunteers; and Coleridge's dreamy estimate that it might take two years to have the first salable section of the dictionary off the presses—for it was to be sold in parts, to help keep revenues coming in—was wrong by a factor of ten. It was this kind of woefully naive underestimate—of work, of time, of money—that at first so hindered the dictionary's advance. No one had a clue what they were up against: They were marching blindfolded through molasses.

And Herbert Coleridge's early death slowed matters down even more. He died after only two years at work, at the age of thirty-one, not even halfway through looking at the quotations of words beginning with A. He had been caught in the rain on the way to a Philological Society lecture, and he had sat through it in the unheated upstairs room on St.

James's Square, caught a chill, and died. His last recorded words were: "I must begin Sanskrit tomorrow."

Furnivall then took over and threw all of his breezy energy and single-minded determination into his work—but in the same madcap, irresponsible manner that had already made him such legions of enemies. He had the bright and enduring idea of hiring a team of subeditors—whom he would interpose between the volunteer readers, now gaily sending in their slips of paper with the necessary quotations—and the editor himself.

The subs could check the incoming slips for accuracy and value, then sort them into bundles, and place them in the pigeonholes. It would then be up to the editor to decide on the word he was going to "do"—take out from its place in the alphabetically arranged pigeonholes the bundle of quotations for that target word, and decide which of the quotations best suited his needs. Which one was the earliest—this was vitally important, of course; and which others, thereafter, demonstrated the slow progress of the word, as its meaning varied over the centuries, up to whatever was its primary meaning now.

But Furnivall presided over a project that, in spite of all of his energies and enthusiasm, started slowly but clearly to die. For some reason, never quite explained, Furnivall had not the ginger to keep the hundreds of volunteers enthused, and so, slowly and steadily, they simply stopped reading, stopped sending in the slips. It seemed to many an insurmountable task. Many in fact sent back their books and the papers that Furnivall had sent them to read—in 1879 alone they had returned *two tons* of material. The dictionary was well and truly stalled, perhaps a victim of its own massive ambition. Furnivall's reports to the society became shorter and shorter, his sculling expeditions with waitresses from the ABC longer and longer. In 1868 the *Athenaeum*, the journal that most closely followed the progress of the work, told its London readers that "the general belief is, the project will not be carried out."

But it did not die. James Murray, it will be remembered, had been a member of the Philological Society since 1869. He had already made a name for himself with publications (on Scottish dialect), with huge editing tasks (of Scottish poetry), and with noble but unfinished projects (such as a planned work on the declension of German nouns). He had left the Chartered Bank of India and had resumed his beloved teaching, this time at the distinguished London public school Mill Hill.

Furnivall—who, though clearly committed to the dictionary, simply lacked the personal qualities necessary to lead it—thought Murray a perfect choice as editor. He approached Murray and others of the society too: Would not this astonishing young man (Murray was then just over forty) not be the ideal candidate? And moreover, would not the Oxford University Press, with its academic distinction, comparatively deep pockets, and a flexible view of literary time, be the ideal house to publish the work?

Murray was persuaded to produce some specimen sheets, suggestions of how the work might look. He chose the words *arrow, carouse, castle,* and *persuade,* and in the late autumn of 1877 the pages were duly sent off to Oxford, to the press's notoriously difficult Delegates—essentially, the board of directors, who were infamous for being dauntingly high-brow, irritatingly pedantic, and fiscally mean. Furnivall continued to meet other publishers and printers—the house of Macmillan was at one time deeply involved, but backed out after a dispute with Furnivall—and made endlessly certain that the big dictionary remained on everybody's mind.

The twin notions of selecting the right editor and the proper publisher continued to vex the lexicographical and commercial literary establishments of England for the final years of the seventies. Oxford's Delegates first dismayed everyone by saying that they cared little for Murray's specimens: They wanted more proof that Murray had looked hard enough for quotations for his four chosen words; they said they didn't like the way he had offered the words' pronunciations; and they dithered about whether or not his etymological section should be omitted (not least because they were already publishing a quite separate and scholarly *Etymological Dictionary* of their own).

In exasperation Murray and Furnivall looked hopefully toward the Cambridge press, but the syndics there (the local equivalent of the Oxford Delegates) offered only a brusque rebuff. Lobbying went on, in common rooms and London clubs, week after week. And as time passed, so Oxford slowly became persuaded that changes could be made, that the powers that be might ultimately find the pages of the proposed book to be acceptable, that Murray might well be the man, and that the big dictionary could in fact one day have the commercial and intellectual appeal that Oxford wanted.

* * *

It was finally, on April 26, 1878, that James Murray was invited up to Oxford for the first meeting with the Delegates themselves. He had come expecting to be terrified of them; they imagined they would be dismissive of him. But to everyone's surprised delight, he found that he rather liked the grand old men who sat in that great Oxford boardroom, and, more to the point, they discovered in short order that they very much liked him. The upshot of the meeting was the Delegates' decision, in a moment of subdued and characteristically Oxonian jubilation—celebrated with a glass or two of indifferent dry sherry—to proceed.

Arguments over the details of the contract—which were often bitter, but were rarely conducted in person by a decidedly other-worldly James Murray (though his hard-headed wife, Ada, did have things to say)—took another full year. Finally, on March 1, 1879, almost a quarter of a century after the speech by Richard Chenevix Trench, a document was formally agreed upon: James Murray was to edit, on behalf of the Philological Society of London, *The New English Dictionary on Historical Principles*, which would spread itself across an estimated seven thousand quarto pages in four thick volumes, and take ten years to complete. It was still a woeful underestimate, but the work was now beginning properly, and this time it was never to stop.

Within days Murray had made two decisions. First, he would build a corrugated iron shed on the grounds of Mill Hill School, he would call it the Scriptorium (the first of his two specially built headquarters), and would edit the great dictionary from there. And second, he would write and have published a four-page appeal—"to the English-speaking and English-reading public"—for a vast fresh corps of volunteers. The committee, he declared, "want help from readers in Great Britain, America and the British Colonies, to finish the volunteer work so enthusiastically commenced twenty years ago, by reading and extracting the books which still remain unexamined."

The four sheets of paper—eight pages of writing—went out to the magazines and newspapers of the day, which regarded them as a press release and published such parts as seemed likely to interest their readers. They went out also to bookshops and newsstands, and assistants handed them to customers. Librarians handed them out as bookmarks, and there were small wooden cases in shops and libraries from which the public could take them and read them. Before long they had found wide circulation all around the United Kingdom and its various dominions, old and new.

And sometime in the early 1880s one copy, at least, left inside a book or slipped between the pages of a learned journal, found its way to one of two large cells on the top floor of Block 2 of the Broadmoor Asylum for the Criminally Insane in Crowthorne, Berkshire. It was read, voraciously, by William Minor, a man for whom books, with which one of his two cells was lined from floor to ceiling, had become a second life.

Doctor Minor had been an inmate at Broadmoor for the

previous eight years. He was deluded, true; but he was a sensitive and intelligent man, a graduate of Yale, and well read and curious. He was, understandably, preternaturally anxious to have something useful to do, something that might occupy the weeks and months and years and decades that stretched without limit—"Until Her Majesty's Pleasure be Known"—before him.

This invitation from a Dr. James Murray of Mill Hill, Middlesex, N.W., it seemed, promised an opportunity for intellectual stimulus—and perhaps even a measure of personal redemption—that was far better than any he could otherwise imagine. He would write, immediately.

He took down paper and a pen, and in a firm hand wrote his address: Broadmoor, Crowthorne, Berks. A perfectly ordinary address. To anyone who did not know any better it was merely a means of describing an ordinary house, in an ordinary village, in a prettily rural royal county just beyond the boundaries of London.

And even if someone outside did know the word *asylum*, the sole definition that was available at the time was quite innocent in its explanation. The meaning was to be found in Johnson's dictionary, naturally: "A place out of which he that has fled to it, may not be taken." An asylum was to Doctor Johnson no more than a sanctuary, a refuge. William Chester Minor was quite content to be seen to write from inside such a place—just so long as no one looked too closely for the deeper and more sinister meaning that the word was then gathering to itself in the hard times of Victorian England.

6

The Scholar in Cell Block Two

Bedlam (be·dləm). Forms: I-3 betleem, 3 beþþleæm, 3–6 beth(e)leem, 4 bedleem, 4–8 bethlem, 6– -lehem, 3–7 bedlem, 5 bedelem, 6 bedleme, 6–7 -lame, 6– bedlam. [ME. *Bedlem* = *Bethlem, Bethlehem*; applied to the Hospital of St. Mary of Bethlehem, in London, founded as a priory in 1247, with the special duty of receiving and entertaining the bishop of St. Mary of Bethlehem, and the canons, etc. of this, the mother church, as often as they might come to England. In 1330 it is mentioned as 'an hospital,' and in 1402 as a hospital for lunatics (Timbs); in 1346 it was received under the protection of the city of London, and on the Dissolution of the Monasteries, it was granted to the mayor and citizens, and in 1547 incorporated as a royal foundation for the reception of lunatics. Thence the modern sense, of which instances appear early in 16th c.]

2. The Hospital of St. Mary of Bethlehem, used as an asylum for the reception and cure of mentally deranged persons; originally situated in Bishopsgate, in 1676 rebuilt near London Wall, and in 1815 transferred to Lambeth. *Jack* or *Tom o' Bedlam*: a madman.

3. By extension: A lunatic asylum, a madhouse.

Minor, William Chester. A thin, pale and sharp-featured man with light sandy-coloured hair, deep-set eyes and prominent cheek bones. He is 38 years old, of superior education, indeed a surgeon, but of no known religion. He weights 10 stone, one pound, and is formally classified as being Dangerous to Others. He was charged with the willful murder of one George Merrett of Lambeth, was found Not Guilty on the Grounds of Insanity. He says he has been the victim of persecution for years—the victim of the lower classes, in whom he has no faith. Persons unknown are trying to injure him, with poison.

So begin the case notes for Broadmoor patient 742, based on an examination conducted in the afternoon of the day he was admitted, Wednesday, April 17, 1872.

Guards had brought him there in shackles, along with another murderer—a man who was classified "Too Insane to be Tried"—named Edmund Dainty: Both had been waiting in jail at Newington in Surrey until the necessary papers had been brought down from London. They were brought first by steam train to the small red-brick Gothic railway station that had been built by and then named for Wellington College, one of the great schools of southern England, which stood nearby. A black Broadmoor landau, its roof closed, then took Minor and his escorts through the narrow, leafy lanes winding around the tiny village. The horses were sweating slightly as they hauled the four-wheel vehicle and its occupants up the low sandstone hill at the top of which stands Broadmoor itself.

The Special Hospital, as it is called today, still looks a forbidding place, even though much of what must have rendered it quite terrifying in Victorian times is now hidden discreetly behind its high, smoothly round-topped, modern maximum-security walls. In 1872 Doctor Minor came to the original front gate—two triple-storied towers with heavily barred windows, with an imposing archway between, topped by a large black-faced clock. The arch was closed by a massive pair of green outer wooden doors. A peephole in one snapped open at the sound of the horses' hooves, the doors swung back to reveal another set of heavy gates, ten yards deeper into the asylum.

The landau moved swiftly inside, the front doors were slammed closed and bolted hard, and the lights in the dim and cavernous reception area were switched on. Doctor Minor was ordered to step out, to be searched. His chains were removed, to be taken back to Surrey. The escorting tipstaff (the Broadmoor bailiff) handed over the papers—a long

warrant in elegant copperplate, above the signature of Henry
Austin Bruce, Her Majesty's Principal Secretary of State for
the Home Department. The asylum superintendent, a kindly
and sympathetic man named William Orange, had his dep-
uty sign the receipt.

Doctor Minor was led through the second set of gates
and into Block 4, the admissions building. He heard the
horses turn around, heard his escort clamber up into the
carriage and order the driver to return to the railway station. He heard the outer gates open to let the carriage out,
and then close again. There was a resounding second crash
as the inner metal gates shut and were bolted and chained.
He was now formally and properly a Broadmoor inmate,
confined in what would probably be his home for the rest
of his natural life.

It was a fairly new home, however. Broadmoor had been open
just nine years. It had been built because the state's main lunatic asylum, the Hospital of St. Mary of Bethlehem—from
which we have the word *bedlam* for a madhouse—was now
full to bursting. (By coincidence, it was located in Lambeth,
less than a mile from the murder site.) Legal recognition of
criminal madness had been established by Parliament in
1800, and judges had for the past half century been dispatch-
ing into asylums—and sentencing to stay there until the
monarch's "Pleasure be Known"—scores of men and women
who would hitherto have been sent to ordinary prisons.

The Victorians, with their characteristic mix of severity and enlightenment, believed the inmates could both

be kept securely away from the public to whom they were so dangerous, and properly treated. But the enlightenment only went so far: While nowadays the Broadmoor inmates are patients, and Broadmoor itself a special hospital, a century ago there was no mincing of words: The inmates were lunatics and criminals, they were treated by "alienists" and "mad-doctors," and Broadmoor was indubitably an asylum, in which they were firmly imprisoned.

Broadmoor certainly looked and felt—and was meant to look and feel—like a prison. It had been designed by a military architect, Sir Joshua Jebb, who had previously created two of England's darkest high-security penitentiaries, Pentonville and Dartmoor. It had long, gaunt cell blocks, severe and intimidating; all the buildings were of dark red brick; all the windows were barred; there was a huge wall topped with iron spikes and broken glass.

The institution slouched crablike, ugly, and forbidding on top of its hill: Villagers would look up toward it and shudder. They tested the escape sirens every Monday morning: The banshee wails that echoed and reechoed across the hills were spine chilling; people said the birds remained silent, frightened, for many minutes afterward.

But Doctor Minor, an American murderer—where to put him? The normal practice, which, to judge from his case notes, was almost certainly followed in Minor's case, was to spend several early days asking the newcomer about himself, and then, if he wanted to discuss it, about the crime that had caused him to be sent there. (One newcomer, asked why he had killed his wife and children, told the superintendent: "I don't know why I am telling you all of this. It's none of your business. As a matter of fact it was none of the judge's business either. It was *a purely family affair* [emphasis added].")

Once that was duly accomplished—it was then standard Broadmoor practice never again to ask about the crime—the superintendent decided which of the six male blocks (there were two others for women, securely fenced off from the men) was most suitable. If the patient was judged suicidal (and his records were thereafter written on pink cards, not white) he was put in a cell in Block 6, where there were extra staff members to observe him all the time; if he was diagnosed epileptic he was put in another cell in the same block, a special cell that had padded walls and a wedge-shaped pillow on which he could not suffocate himself during a fit.

If he was thought to be dangerous and violent, he was also shut up in Block 6, or maybe the slightly smaller-staffed Block 1—the two being known variously as the "strong blocks," "the disturbed blocks," or more recently the "refractory blocks." Then as now the two buildings, grimmer and gaunter than the rest, were known among the inmates as the "back blocks," because they have no view over the landscape. They are secure, tough, miserable.

After the first few days of interrogations the Broadmoor doctors realized that their new charge—a doctor himself, after all—was neither epileptic, nor liable to kill himself, nor sufficiently violent to do anyone an injury. So he was sent to Block 2—a relatively comfortable wing that was usually kept for parole patients. It was called the "swell block," the word used in the British sense, meaning it tended to be occupied by swells. A visitor once wrote that Block 2 had an atmosphere "described by someone familiar with both, as identical with that at the Athenaeum Club." It is difficult to imagine that too many members of this most genteel of London's gentlemen's clubs, which included on its rolls most of the bishops and learned men of the land, were thrilled by the comparison.

Yet Minor was made more than just tolerably comfortable—not least because he was a well-born, well-educated man. And he had an income: All the Broadmoor officials knew he was a retired soldier, with a regular army pension paid from the United States. So he was given not one cell but two, a pair of connecting rooms at the south end of the block's top floor. The rooms were kept unlocked by day; at night any medicines and food he might need were handed in through a long vertical slot, too narrow for an arm to reach out, with a lockable door on its outer side.

The windows had iron bars on the inside—but to compensate there was an enchanting view: a long shallow valley of cattle-filled meadows with the cows standing in the shadow of great oak trees; the Broadmoor tennis courts and a small cricket ground to one side; a line of low blue hills crowned with beeches in the distance. On that early spring day, with clear skies and lilacs and apple blossom and the songs of larks and thrushes, perhaps the sentence may not have seemed altogether a nightmare.

At the north end of the corridor sat the guard—known at the asylum as an attendant—who kept watch over the twenty men on his floor. He had keys, presided over the ever-locked door to the floor itself, and would let them in and out of their rooms to visit the bathroom; and during the day he kept a small gas flame burning, from a brass jet beside him. The men were not allowed matches: This is where they came to light their cigarettes or their pipes, from the tobacco ration they were handed each week. (The tobacco all came from H.M. Customs service: Anything confiscated as contraband at the ports was handed over to the Home Office for distribution at the prisons and the state lunatic asylums.)

Within days the American vice-consul was writing, making sure that the hapless army officer was being well looked after. Might it be possible for "our poor friend," he prayed, to have some of his personal effects sent down? (They had been left at the consulate to help pay any of the diplomats' expenses at court.) Is it in theory possible to visit? To cheer him up, could we send him a pound of Dennis's coffee and some French plums? Mr. Orange was silent on the specific matter of plums, but told the consul that Doctor Minor could have whatever he liked so long as it didn't prejudice his safety or the asylum's disciplined running.

So a week later the official sent up a leather portmanteau by rail: It held a frock coat and three waistcoats, three pairs of drawers and four undervests, four shirts, four collars, six pocket handkerchiefs, a prayer book, a box of photographs, four pipes, cigarette papers, a bag of tobacco, a map of London, a diary, and a fob watch and gold chain—the last a family heirloom, it had been said during the trial.

Most important of all, the superintendent reported later, the doctor was given back his drawing materials: a cheap deal drawing box and its contents, a paintbox and a collection of pens, a drawing board, sketchbooks, and painting cards. He would now be able to occupy his time constructively, which all patients were encouraged to do.

Over the succeeding months Minor furnished his cells comfortably—much, indeed, as a member of the Athenaeum might. He had money: His officer's pension of about twelve hundred dollars a year was paid to his brother Alfred in Connecticut—he acted for William, whom the state had designated "an incapable person"—who regularly telegraphed funds to England to keep his sick brother's running account up-to-date. Using this constant credit, Doctor Minor satiated his one consuming passion: books.

He demanded first that his own books be sent over from home in New Haven. Once they were installed he ordered, from the big London bookstores, scores upon scores of new and secondhand volumes, which he first stacked in precarious piles in his cells until he asked—and paid for—bookshelves to be built. In the end he had converted the more westerly of the two rooms into a library, with a writing desk, a couple of chairs, and floor-to-ceiling teak bookshelves.

He kept his easel and his paints in the other, easterly room; he also kept a small selection of wines and some bourbon, with which the consul kept him supplied. He took up the flute again, and gave lessons to some of his neighbor inmates. He also found that he was permitted—and was well able to afford—to pay one of his fellow patients to perform work for him—tidying his room, sorting his books, cleaning up after a painting session. Life, which in those first months had been at least tolerable, now started to become really quite

agreeable: William Minor was able to live a life of total leisure and security, he was warm and reasonably well fed, his
health was attended to, he could stroll along the long gravel
pathway known as the Terrace, he could take his ease on one
of the benches by the lawn and gaze at the shrubbery, or he
could read and paint to his heart's content.

His cells still exist—not much at Broadmoor has changed
in a century, and although Block 2 is now called Essex House,
it is still much preferred for those patients who are in for the
long haul. One of the two rooms—the westerly of the pair,
where Doctor Minor maintained his library—houses a patient whose violent propensities are readily apparent: The
room is littered with magazines devoted to bodybuilding,
posters on the wall celebrate the achievements of Rambo-
like figures, there are technical drawings of large American
motorcycles, and a slogan torn from a comic book has been
pasted onto the cell door. It says: Mad Killer.

The other room, where Minor painted, was by contrast
so tidy that it looked almost unoccupied: The bed was so well
made that one could have bounced the proverbial coin on its
taut surface, leather shoes were neatly arranged and polished,
clothes were hanging neatly in the wardrobe. There were no
books, nothing on the walls. The fireplace had long since
been boarded up, although there was a mantel, which had a
small desk calendar. The room's occupant, I was told, was an
Egyptian.

Doctor Minor's sanity, or lack thereof, was never in
doubt. He was never so ill as to be ordered away from the

benign atmosphere of Block 2 and into the harsher regime of the back blocks (though a strange and terrible incident in 1902 did take him away from his rooms for many weeks). But the ward notes show that his delusions became over the years ever more fixed, ever more bizarre, and that there seemed no likelihood that he would ever regain his reasoning. He was comfortable in Broadmoor, maybe; but there was nowhere else he could be allowed to live.

The ward notes from his first ten years show the sad and relentless progress of his downward spiral. Already at the time he was admitted he had a detailed awareness of the curious happenings that plagued him at night—always at night. Small boys, he believed, were put up in the rafters above his bed; they came down when he was fast asleep, chloroformed him, and then forced him to perform indecent acts—though whether with them as boys, or whether with the women of whom he dreamed constantly, the record-keepers were never clear. He claimed he would awaken with abrasions around his nose and mouth where they had clamped the gas bottle; the bottoms of his pajama legs were always damp, he said, indicating he had been forced to walk in a stupor through the night.

April 1873: "Dr. Minor is thin and anaemic, excitable in manner, though appears rational by day and occupies himself with painting and playing the flute. But at night he barricades the door of his room with furniture, and connects the handle of the door with the furniture using a piece of string, so that he will awaken if anyone tries to enter the bedroom. . . ."

June 1875: "The doctor is convinced that intruders manage to get in—from under the floor, or through the windows—and that they pour poison into his mouth through a funnel: he now insists on being weighed each morning to see if the poison has made him heavier."

August 1875: "The expression of his face in the morning is often haggard and wild, as though he did not obtain much rest. He complains that he feels as if a cold iron has been pressed against his teeth at night, and that something is being pumped into him. Otherwise, no change."

A year later the demons were seeming to have a depressing influence. In February 1876 the doctors noted: "A fellow-patient stated today that Dr. Minor came to see him in the Boot Room and said he would give him everything, if only he would cut his—Dr. Minor's—throat. An Attendant was ordered to look after him."

The following year was no better. "Socially," he was reported as explaining to an attendant in May 1877, "all systems are based on schemes of corruption and knavery, and he is the subject of their machinations. This lies at the heart of the brutal torture to which he is subjected each night. His spinal marrow is pierced and his heart is operated on with instruments of torture. His assailants come through the floor. . . ."

In 1878 technology becomes a part of the villainy. "Electric currents from unseen sources are passed through his body, he insists. Electric buttons are placed on his forehead, he is placed in a wagon and trundled across the countryside." He was taken as far afield as Constantinople, he told an attendant once, where he is made to perform lewd acts in public. "They are," he declared, "trying to make a pimp of me!"

But while the delusions clearly persisted and worsened over those early asylum years, the clinical notes do show—and crucially to this story—the parallel development of a more thoughtful and scholarly side to the afflicted man.

"With the exception of his impressions on the subject of his night-time visitations," says one entry in the late 1870s, "he talks very coherently and intelligently on most topics. He works in his bit of garden, and is fairly cheerful just now—but he has his days of moodiness and reserve." A year later a doctor records simply: "He is rational and intelligent for the most part,"

He also begins to settle down, starting to regard the great hospital as his home and the attendants as his family. "He is not particularly aware that he is anxious to go back to America, as at one time he was," writes another doctor. "All he asks is a little bit more freedom, perhaps to go and see sights in London, or perhaps visit the orchid show for which he had just received a card." Yet the doctor who conducted this particular interview was certain of his patient's condition, and inscribed a sentence which seems in hindsight almost to have sealed William Minor's eternal fate.

There can be no doubt that Dr. Minor, though on occasion very calm and collected, is generally-speaking more abundantly insane, and shows himself to be more so, than he was some years ago. He has the calm and firm conviction that he is almost

nightly the victim of torment and purposive annoy-
ance, on the parts of the Attendants and others connected with an infernal criminal scheme.

It was at about this time that there came two developments, one of which by chance led indirectly to the other. The
first stemmed from a factor that is not uncommon among
those who commit appalling crimes: Minor became truly re-
morseful for what he had done, and resolved to try and make
some kind of amends. It was with this in mind that he took
the bold step of writing to his victim's widow, via the American Embassy, which he knew had helped raise a fund for her
in the months immediately following the tragedy.

He explained to Eliza Merrett how immeasurably sorry
he was for what he had done, and he offered to try to help
in any way he could—perhaps by settling money on her or
her children. Already Minor's stepmother, Judith, had contributed: Now, perhaps, and if Mrs. Merrett would only be so
gracious as to accept, he could do rather more.

The letter seems to have worked a small miracle: Not
only did Mrs. Merrett agree to accept financial help from
Minor—she also asked if it might be possible to visit him.
It was an unprecedented request, that an incarcerated murderer be allowed to spend time with a relative of his victim;
but the Home Office, after discussing the matter with Doctor
Orange, agreed to one experimental supervised visit. Accord-
ingly, sometime during late 1879, Mrs. Eliza Merrett traveled
up from Lambeth to Broadmoor and first met the man who
had ended her husband's life seven years before, and who had

so drastically changed her own life and the lives of her seven children.

The meeting, according to Doctor Orange's notes, was at first tense, but it progressed well, and by its end Mrs. Merrett had agreed to come again. Before long she was making monthly ventures down to Crowthorne, eager to talk with interested sympathy to this now seemingly harmless American. And though the conversations apparently stopped short of developing into any real friendship, it is believed that she made Minor an offer that was to lead to the second of the major developments of this period of his life. She agreed, it seems, to bring parcels of books to Minor from the antiquarian dealers in London.

Eliza Merrett knew very little of books—indeed, she was barely literate. But when she saw how keenly Doctor Minor collected and cherished his old volumes, and when she listened to his querulous remarks about the delays and costs of the postal service between London and Crowthorne, she made an offer to collect his orders for him, and bring them down on her visits. And so it happened that, month after month, Mrs. Merrett began delivering packages, wrapped in brown paper and sealed with twine and wax, from the West End's great book emporiums, like Maggs, Bernard Quaritch, and Hatchards.

The delivery system, such as it was, probably remained in place for only a few months—Mrs. Merrett eventually took to drink and apparently lost all interest in the curious and eccentric unfortunate. But the system appears during its brief life to have led what was undeniably the most serendipitous event in William Minor's otherwise melancholy life.

For it was in the early 1880s that he stumbled across the first of James Murray's famous appeals for volunteers, which asked for interested parties to indicate that they might be prepared to work on the new dictionary. Murray first published his appeal in April 1879 and had two thousand copies printed and circulated by booksellers: One would almost certainly have found its way, probably fairly soon after its distribution, into one or more of the packages that Mrs. Merrett brought to Minor at the asylum.

The eight pages explained in very broad terms what was likely to be wanted. First there were Murray's own suggestions for the kind of books that needed to be read:

> In the Early English period up to the invention of Printing so much has been done and is doing that little outside help is needed. But few of the earliest printed books—those of Caxton and his successors—have yet been read, and any one who has the opportunity and time to read one or more of these, either in the originals, or accurate reprints, will confer valuable assistance by so doing. The later sixteenth-century literature is very fairly done; yet here several books remain to be read. The seventeenth century, with so many more writers, naturally shows still more unexplored territory. The nineteenth-century books, being within the reach of everyone, have been read widely; but a large number remain unrepresented, not only of those published

during the last ten years while the Dictionary has been in abeyance, but also of earlier date. But it is in the eighteenth century above all that help is urgently needed. The American scholars promised to get the eighteenth-century literature taken up in the United States, a promise which they appear not to have any extent fulfilled, and we must now appeal to English readers to share the task, for nearly the whole of that century's books, with the exception of Burke's works, have still to be gone through.

After this Murray listed rather more than two hundred specific authors whose works, in his view, were essential reading. The list was quite awesome: Most of the volumes were rare, and likely to be in the hands of only a very few collectors. Some books, on the other hand, were already available at Murray's newly established dictionary library at Mill Hill: They could be sent to readers who promised to do work on them. (And vouched to return them: When Henry Furnivall had been editor he found that a number of disgruntled readers used the lending scheme as a means of swelling their own library collections, and neither sent in the requested quotation slips nor ever returned the books.)

Doctor Minor was clearly in one of his more scholarly, reflective, and positive moods when he read the pamphlet, for he responded with alacrity and enthusiasm. He wrote to James Murray almost immediately, formally volunteering his services as a reader.

It is not wholly clear, though, just when this was—not

clear exactly when Minor first started his legendary work. Murray recalled later that he had received Minor's letter "very soon after I commenced the Dictionary." No correspondence between the doctor and the dictionary has been traced, however, until 1885—which is hardly "very soon."

But one clue exists: There had been an article in the *Athenaeum* magazine in September 1879, suggesting that Americans might like to become more keenly involved, and it is quite probable that Minor, who is known to have subscribed to the magazine in Broadmoor, would have seen it. Based on this assumption, on Murray's recollections, and on the records of Minor's contributions that have lately been unearthed in the Bodleian Library at Oxford, it seems probable that his relationship with the dictionary got under way in 1880 or 1881.

But where did Murray think his correspondent was living, and what did he think he did? Murray told his correspondent that he remembered only that the first and subsequent letters from Minor had been addressed to the dictionary office simply from "Broadmoor, Crowthorne, Berkshire." Murray was too busy to ruminate on the matter, no matter how curiously familiar the address might have been. By the time he read Minor's first letter he had already received about eight hundred similar letters in response to his appeal—he was being swamped by the success of his entreaty.

He replied to Minor with his characteristic courtesy, saying that on the basis of his apparent qualifications, enthusiasm, and interest he should start reading immediately, going through any of the volumes he might already have, or else looking to the dictionary office for copies of books he might require.

In due course, Murray continued, the doctor could expect to receive particular word requests—in the particular event that the dictionary editors had trouble finding quotations for a specific word on their own. For the time being, however, Doctor Minor and all the other early respondents, to whom the editor expressed his "considerable gratitude," should just start reading and should start making word lists and writing quotations in a careful, systematic, but general way.

Two additional sheets of printed paper Murray was enclosing with the letter, which underlined a formal agreement that Doctor Minor had been officially welcomed as a volunteer reader, would offer any necessary further advice.

But through all this, James Murray explained some years later, "I never gave a thought to who Minor might be. I thought he was either a practicing medical man of literary tastes with a good deal of leisure, or perhaps a retired medical man or surgeon who had no other work."

The truth about his new American correspondent was a great deal stranger than this detached, innocent, and otherworldly Scotsman could have ever imagined.

7

Entering the Lists

catchword (kæ·tʃwɒɹd). [f. CATCH- 3 b + WORD.]

1. *Printing.* The first word of the following page inserted at the right-hand lower corner of each page of a book, below the last line. (Now rarely used.)

2. A word so placed as to catch the eye or attention; *spec.* **a.** the word standing at the head of each article in a dictionary or the like;

1879 *Directions to Readers for Dict.*, Put the word as a catchword at the upper corner of the slip. **1884** *Athenæum* 26 Jan. 124/2 The arranging of the slips collected . . . and the development of the various senses of every Catchword.

The two small closely printed sheets that came as an addendum to Murray's first letter turned out to be a set of meticulously worded instructions. When his morning mail was delivered by the ward staff that day, Minor must have fallen upon this one envelope eagerly, reading and rereading its contents. But it was not the content alone that fascinated him: A list of rules for dictionary helpers was not the cause of his excitement.

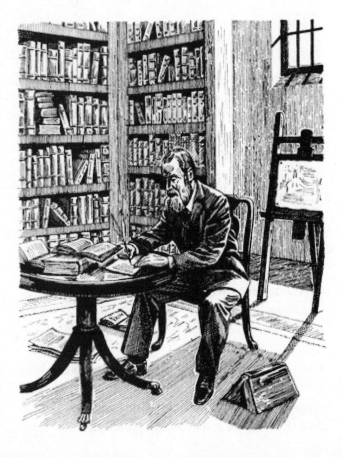

It was the simple fact that they had been sent to him in the first place. The letter from James Murray represented, in Minor's view, a token of the further forgiveness and understanding that Eliza Merrett's visits to him had already suggested. The invitation seemed a long-sought badge of renewed membership in the society from which he had been so long estranged. By being sent these sheets of rules he was, he felt, being received back into a corner of the real world. A corner that admittedly was still housed in a pair of cells in an alien madhouse—but one that had firmly forged links to the world of learning, and connections with a more comfortable reality.

After a decade of languishing in the dark slough of imprisonment, intellectual isolation, and remove, Minor felt that at last he was being hoisted back up onto the sunlit uplands of scholarship. And with what he saw as this reenlistment in the ranks, so Minor's self-worth began, at least marginally, to reemerge, to begin seeping back. From the little evidence that survives in his medical records, he appears to have started recovering his confidence and even his contentment, both with every moment that he spent reading Murray's acceptance letter, and then when he prepared to embark on his self-set task.

For a while at least he seemed truly happier. Even the sternly worded Victorian ward notes of the day hint that the temper of this usually suspicious, broody, prematurely elderly-looking middle-aged man (he was now approaching fifty) had somehow started to turn. His personality was undergoing, even if only for a short while, a sea change—and all because, at long last, he had something valuable to do.

Yet in its very value lay a problem, as Minor saw it. The doctor swiftly came to realize, and was daunted by the realization, the simple fact that this great work's immense potential value to history, to posterity, and to the English-speaking world meant that it had to be done properly. Murray's papers had explained that the dictionary was all about the gathering of hundreds of thousands of quotations. It was a task that was almost unimaginably vast. Could it be done, from an asylum cell?

Minor was both wise enough to understand and ask himself the question (since he knew well where he was, and why he was there) and then, in a partial answer, to applaud Murray for having taken the right approach to the work on which he was about to embark. Minor's own love of books and literature gave him some knowledge of dictionaries, and an appreciation of what was good and what not so good about those that had already been published. So on reflection he decided that he very much wanted to work for the project, and to be a part of it—not solely because it would give him something worthwhile to do, which was his first reason, but mainly because in his opinion Murray's plan for doing it was so self-evidently right.

But Murray's plan meant that there was clearly going to be much more to his cellbound duties than the mere enjoyment of a blissful and leisured romp through the history of published English literature. Minor needed now to pay absolutely scrupulous regard to what he read, to trawl religiously for whatever happened to be needed by Murray's team, and eventually to select from the cod of his net the very best possible entries to send away to be included in the book.

Murray's notes showed him how best this might be done. The quotations, said the editor's first page, were to be written on half sheets of writing paper. The target word—the "catchword," as Murray liked to call it—was to be written at the top left. The crucial date of the quotation should be written just below it, then the name of the author and title of the cited book, the page number, and finally, the full text of the sentence being quoted. Preprinted slips had already been prepared for some books that were important, well known, and likely to be used a great deal, familiar works by such as Chaucer, Dryden, Hazlett, and Swift—readers assigned to these books needed only write to Mill Hill to have some sent; otherwise, Murray asked them to please write out their own slips in full, arrange them alphabetically, and send them on to the Scriptorium.

All this was simple enough. But, everyone wanted to ask—just what words were to be sought out?

Murray's early rules were clear and unambiguous: *Every* word was a possible catchword. Volunteers should try to find a quotation for each and every word in a book. They should perhaps concentrate their efforts on words that struck them as rare, obsolete, old-fashioned, new, peculiar, or used in a peculiar way; but they should also look assiduously for ordinary words as well, providing that the sentence that included it said something about the use or meaning of the word. Special attention also needed to be paid to words that seemed to be new or tentative, obsolete or archaic, so that the date could be used to help fix the moment of their introduction into the language. All that, Murray hoped, was surely plain enough.

But then again, asked would-be readers—how many quotations should be supplied for each word? "As many as convenient," Murray wrote back, especially where different contexts tended either to explain differences in the meaning or helped to illustrate the subtle variations in a particular word's usage. The more quotation slips that came in to the iron shed he had built in Mill Hill, the better: He assured readers that he had an ample supply of assistants to sort them, and that his floors had been especially strengthened to hold them.

(More than two tons of slips of papers had already come in from Coleridge and Furnivall's first efforts, Murray added. But he didn't allow as to how many of them had been nibbled at by mice or ruined by damp, nor did he reveal that one batch was found in a baby's bassinet, or that a load of slips beginning with the letter *I* had been left in a broken-bottomed hamper in an empty vicarage, or that the entire letter *F* had been accidentally sent off to Florence, or that thousands of slips were so poorly handwritten that, Murray reported to a friend, it would have made for easier reading if they had been written in Chinese.)

The second sheet of notes seemed to Minor at first to offer rather more practical, if much more prosaic, help. It first made clear that Murray had a fund from which he could repay the postage to those volunteers who sent packages of slips but could not afford to do so; and it asked that the packages be sent to Mill Hill by book post, with their ends unsealed, so that Murray didn't have to pay fines for those that had been shut with even the tiniest bit of adhesive (forbidden by Post Office regulations).

Many early readers turned out to be dreadfully confused; they simply did not understand the scope of their allotted task. For example, asked a couple of them, Did every single use of the word *the* within any one book require an illustrative quote? There would be tens of thousands from any volume, before any of the substantive words were even begun. And further, wailed one of the women readers, what if one had plowed through all 750 pages of a volume, as she just had, and found not a single rare word to extract?

Murray's notes offer a tolerant and genial-enough response to this kind of complaint, though a faint sense of his Calvinist asperity glimmers between the lines. No, he spoke through moderately gritted teeth, there was really no need to offer scores of illustrations for definite articles and prepositions, unless the circumstances turned out to be very strange. And no, no, *no!* books were *not* to be scoured for rare words alone—he had to remind volunteers of this fact time and again. Readers must find and note *all and any* words that seemed interesting, or that were quoted in interesting and signifying ways or in ways that were *good, apt,* or *pithy.*

As an example of the dangers of the process so far, he said, he had received no fewer than fifty quotes for the word *abusion* (which means "perversion of the truth"), but had had only five for the much more common word *abuse.*

"My editors have to search for precious hours for quotations for examples of ordinary words, which readers disregarded, thinking them not worthy of including," he wrote. Think simple, Murray kept insisting: Think simple.

And then, half exasperated that he evidently still hadn't been clear enough, he laid down a distilled version of his instruction, a golden rule, a sentence that was to become the dictionary readers' epigraph. He wanted readers simply to be able to say: "This is a capital quotation for, say, *heaven*, or *half*, or *hug*, or *handful*; it illustrates the meaning or use of the word; it is a suitable instance for the Dictionary." Follow that kind of thinking, Murray insisted, and you will not go too far wrong.

William Minor read and clearly understood all of this. He looked about his library-cell, scanning the volumes in the astonishing collection that he had already accumulated over the previous ten years. He took out the list of books that had come with Murray's original pamphlet. He would see first if he had any on his shelves that might in time become useful.

All of a sudden his books, which had hitherto been merely a fond decoration and a means of letting his mind free itself from the grim routines of Broadmoor life, had become his most precious possession. For the time being at least he could set aside his imaginings about the harm that people were trying to inflict on him and his person: It was instead his hundreds of books that now needed to be kept safe, and away from the predators with whom he believed the asylum to be infested. His books, and his work on the words he found in them, were about to become the defining feature of his newly chosen life. For the next twenty years he would do almost nothing at Broadmoor except enfold himself and his tortured brain in the world of his books, their writings, and their words.

He was maverick enough, original-minded enough, however, to realize that he could do better than simply follow Murray's orders to the letter. Given his peculiar position, his leisure, his library, he could do more, do otherwise. It took him some days of pondering exactly how he might best serve the project; but after some weeks of thinking he came up with what he thought was the best way to tackle the task. He made a decision. He took down from his shelves the first of his books, and laid it open flat on his reading desk.

We cannot be sure which book it was. For sake of illustration, though, let us say the first volume, and which we know he had and used, was a leather-bound, gold-and-marble-edged translation of a French book called *Complete Woman*, by one Jacques du Boscq. Published in London in 1639, it had been translated by a man identified only as "N.N."

His arguments for starting with this in particular, and indeed for reading it at all, were many. It was a good seventeenth-century work, it was obscure and exotic, it was filled no doubt with strange and amusing words. After all, Murray had exhorted his volunteers to examine this specific period of literary history: "The seventeenth century, with so many more writers, naturally shows still more unexplored territory." Du Boscq's book, in its anonymous translation, fitted the bill splendidly.

So Minor took from a drawer four sheets of white paper and a bottle of black ink, and he selected a pen with the very finest nib. He folded the paper into a quire, a booklet eight pages thick. Then, with perhaps one last glance down from his cell window at the lush countryside below, he settled in to read his chosen book, line by line, paragraph by paragraph, with slow and infinitely measured care. As he did so, he began a routine that he had planned during his early days of preparation.

Each and every time he found a word that piqued his interest he wrote it down, in tiny, almost microscopic letters, in its proper position in the quire he had made.

The unique manner of his procedure was soon to become a hallmark of Minor's astonishing accuracy and eye for detail. His work would win the admiration and awe of all who were later to see it; even today the quires preserved in the dictionary archives are such as to make people gasp.

Let us choose as an example the moment when he came across the word *buffoon*. He was first struck by the significance of its appearance, in a suitably illustrative sentence, on du Boscq's page 34. He promptly wrote it down in his tiny, perfectly neat, perfectly legible handwriting, on the first page of his blank booklet. He wrote it in the first column, and decided to place the word and its page number in the column about a third of the way down.

The placement was precise, and it was carefully chosen. The reason for this was Minor's certainty that sooner or later he would find another interesting word beginning with the same letter, *b*; that there was a very good chance it would have to be put before *buffoon* and only a very much slimmer chance that it would need to be put after (because with *buffoon*'s second letter being *u*, there were only three possibilities—finding a further word or words whose second letter was again *u*, or one with the only other legitimate second letters, *w*—with only one word,*bwana*—or *y*).

Sure enough, a few pages later he came across the interesting word *balk*, with a nice quotation, and so deserving to be entered in the quire. He placed it on the list above *buffoon*, but with enough space in the event that another *b* word came along whose second letter was somewhere in the alphabet between the new *a* and the old *u*. Five pages further on he then sighted with some pleasure the word *blab*—a word of the very kind he had anticipated—and so in it went, levered into the space that he had so artfully retained below *balk* and well above *buffoon*.

And thus did the wordlist for the first of Doctor Minor's cellful of books begin—word after word after word, each one with its spelling exact, its location in the quire perfectly appropriate, the page number where it was to be found in the source-book precise. From *atom* and *azure*, to *gust* and *hearten, fix* and *foresight*, the list went on and on. Some of the words occurred many times—*feel*, for example, which Minor recorded as cropping up on sixteen of du Boscq's pages, although some of these turned out to be *feeling*, either the gerund (as in "I can't help feeling this way"), or the noun (as with "The feeling of which you speak is painful").

It must have taken him many weeks, perhaps months, to complete this first word list. Perhaps it was well into the year

1883 by the time he had finished it. But even though fully four years had now elapsed since James Murray had sent out his first appeal pamphlet, and more than three years since the first nudge to American readers in the *Athenaeum* magazine, and a year, maybe two, since Minor had read one or other of the appeals and had decided to become involved, he still had not sent one single quotation slip down to the Scriptorium. For all the staff of the dictionary knew, he had lost interest, become overwhelmed, dropped out.

But nothing could have been further from the truth. Doctor Minor in fact had quite another plan of attack—a working method that turned out to be very different from that of all other volunteer readers, but that soon marked him as uniquely valuable in the making of the great dictionary.

For once he had completed the monumental task of writing his first word list from his first book, he replaced that volume and took down another. Perhaps his next was Francis Junius, *The Painting of the Ancients*, from 1638, or Thomas Wilson's *The Rule of Reason*, from 1551. Or perhaps something quite different. It could have been any one of hundreds of books, for he had a prodigious collection, and it would be his practice to select one, then another, and then yet another and write a new word list for each one. One book might take him three months to complete, in the kind of detail he felt his distant editors would demand.

And so he would work away, day after day—the tiny spy window in his door clicking open and shut every hour or so from the outside as the Broadmoor attendants checked on the safety and the existence of their strange patient. He would be

working hard, deep in thought and with rapt concentration:
He would index and collect and collate words and sentences
from each of the books, until his prison desk was heavy with
the quires of paper, each one containing a master list of the
indexed words from his eclectic, very valuable, and much val-
ued little gem of a library.

Although we cannot be sure which of his books he read first,
we do know the titles of some of the books that he did read.
Most of them, it turns out, reflect his keenly forlorn interest in
travel and history. One can only imagine how his poor mind
must have raced, trapped as it was in his book-lined retreat
on the top floor of his cell block. How frustrated and pinioned
he must have felt, reading line after line of such books as the
one by Thomas Herbert, written in 1634, titled *A Relation of
Some Yeares Travaile Begunne Anno 1626 into Afrique and the
Greater Asia*; one can only suspect how homesick Minor must
have felt for Trincomalee (and his native girls) on reading
and indexing Nicholas Lichfield's 1582 translation of Fernão
Lopez de Castanheda's *First Booke of the Historie of the Dis-
coverie and Conquest of the East Indies*.

One by one his collection of carefully assembled word
leaflets mounted up. By the autumn of 1884 he had enough
of them, a large-enough selection of words for which he had
readily accessible quotations, to begin inquiring of the dictionary editors—and Murray himself in particular—which
catchwords, precisely, were then needed. For while all the
other volunteers would simply read their assigned books,
note down interesting quotations on their slips of paper as

they came across them and send them off in bundles, Doctor Minor, with all the time on his hands, was able to extrapolate on his radically different, homegrown approach.

With his rapidly growing collection of word lists and his indexes, he stood ready now to help the dictionary project as it needed to be helped, by sending over quotations at the precise time the editors needed them. He could keep up; he could be abreast of the progress of the dictionary all the while, because he had ready access to the words that were needed, when they were wanted. He had made a key, a Victorian word-Rolodex, a dictionary within a dictionary, and it was instantly available. The quires of lists on his plain wooden table represented an accumulated creation of which he was quite rightly and jealously proud.

His practice was first to write to the dictionary and ask what letter or what word was being worked on. Then, on receiving a reply, he would refer to his own index quires to see if he had already noted down the wanted word. If he had—and given his method and his wide and energetic reading it was more than likely that he had—he would follow his own notation of the page number or numbers, and go straight to the word's appearance or appearances in one of his books. Then, and only then, he would transcribe the best sentence containing the word onto a readymade quotation slip and send it directly to the Scriptorium.

It was an unprecedented approach—the kind of technique that only someone with an immense amount of energy and disposable time could contemplate. And of course it was a technique that suited the editors famously: They knew now that down at this mysteriously anonymous address in Crowthorne, in all probability they had on tap, as it were, a supply of fully indexed words together with their associated citations and quotations.

With the arrival of Minor's first letter, saying what he had done and how ready he was for further inquiry, Murray's hard-pressed staff discovered that life had become in theory very much simpler. From this moment forward they were not obliged only to ferret through their shelves and pigeonholes, and to trawl through thousands of existing slips for quotations that might or might not exist for a word they wanted to include. They could simply decide on a word that was giving them problems, write to Crowthorne, and ask for it.

With good fortune—and with a high statistical likelihood—they would in due course receive a letter and a package from Doctor Minor, giving the precise chapter and verse for whatever was wanted, enclosing the quotation slips at the very instant they were needed to be pasted onto a page for the compositors, the typesetters and the printers.

The first word to be tried in this way was a deceptively simple one (to the extent that any individual word is simple compared to any other). It was a word that was due to be included in the dictionary's second fascicle, or part, being readied to be printed and published in the later summer of 1885. Please inspect your word lists, wrote a subeditor, to see if you can find in them references to the word *art*, and to all its derived forms.

The letter went directly to Doctor Minor at Broadmoor, as his invitational letter had suggested. Whichever of Murray's subeditors first asked him the question in reply had no ideas about the man from whom an answer was sought. For many years thence no one in the Scriptorium was to learn anything about him, except for the undeniable truth that he was very good at his job, very quick, and on his way to becoming an indispensable member of the great new dictionary team.

Art was to be his first test.

8

Annulated, Art, Brick-Tea, Buckwheat

Poor (pū^əɹ), *a. (sb.)* Forms: *a.* 3–5 pouere (povere), 3–6 pouer (pover), (4 poeuere, poeure, pouir), 4–5 poer, powere, 5 poyr, 5–6 power, (6 poware). *β* 3–5 poure, 4–6 powre, pour. *γ.* 3–7 (–9 *dial.*) pore, 4–7 poore, (6) 7– poor. *δ. Sc.* and *north. dial.* 4–6 pur, 4–8 pure, (4 puyre, 5 pwyr, poyr, 6 peur(e, pwir, puire), 6– puir(ü), (9 peer). [ME. *pov(e)re, pouere, poure*, a. OF. *povre, -ere, poure*, in mod.F. *pauvre*, dial. *paure, pouvre, poure* = Pr. *paubre, paure*, It. *povero*, Sp., Pg. *pobre*:-L. *pauper*, late L. also *pauper-us*, poor. The mod.Eng. *poor* and Sc. *puir* represent the ME. *pōre*: with mod. vulgar *pore*, cf. *whore* and the pronunciation of *door, floor*.

On account of the ambiguity of the letter *u* and its variant *v* before 1600, it is uncertain whether ME. *pouere, poure, pouer*, meant *pou-* or *pov-*. The phonetic series *paupere(m, paupre, paubre, pobre, povre*, shows that *povre* preceded *poure*, which may have been reached in late OF., and is the form

in various mod.F. dialects. But the 15th and early
16th c. literary Fr. form was *povre*, artificially spelt
in 15th c. *pauvre*, after L. *pauper*, and ME. *pōre*
(the source of mod.Eng. *poor*) seems to have been
reduced from *povre* like *o'er* from *over, lord* from
loverd. Cf. also POORTITH, PORAIL, POVERTY. But
some Eng. dialects now have *pour* (paur), which
prob. represents ME. *pour* (pūr).]

I. 1. Having few, or no, material possessions;
wanting means to procure the comforts, or the
necessaries, of life; needy, indigent, destitute; *spec.*
(esp. in legal use) so destitute as to be dependent upon gifts or allowances for subsistence. In
common use expressing various degrees, from absolute want to straitened circumstances or limited
means relatively to station, as 'a poor gentleman',
'a poor professional man, clergyman, scholar,
clerk', etc. The opposite of *rich*, or *wealthy*. *Poor
people*, the poor as a class: often with connotation
of humble rank or station.

6. Such, or so circumstanced, as to excite one's
compassion or pity; unfortunate, hapless. Now
chiefly *colloq.*

In many parts of England regularly said of the
dead whom one knew; = late, deceased.

The first slips of snow white unlined paper, six inches by four, and covered with William Minor's neat, elaborately cursive, and so distinctively American handwriting in greenish black ink, began to drift out from the Broadmoor post room in the spring of 1885. By the late summer they were arriving at their destination in small brown paper packets every month, and then larger packets every week. Before long the gentle shower of paper had turned into a raging blizzard, one that was to howl up from Crowthorne unceasingly for almost all of the next twenty years.

The paper slips were not, however, sent to Mill Hill. By the time Doctor Minor had begun to engage in the second stage of his work, contributing the quotations rather than amassing the lists, James Murray and his team had all moved up to Oxford. The editor had been persuaded to give up his comfortable job as a schoolteacher, and despite the poor pay and the interminable hours, he had taken the plunge into full-time lexicography.

This was in spite of a general mood of malaise and wretchedness. Murray's experiences with the first years of work on the big dictionary were far from happy, and many were the times he had vowed to resign. The Delegates at the Press were parsimonious and interfering; the pace of work was proving insufferably slow; his health was suffering from the interminable hours, his monomaniacal devotion to an almost impossible task.

But then there was one sustaining fact: The first of the

fascicles, the revenue-producing installments into which Oxford insisted that the dictionary be divided, had at last been published, on January 29, 1884. Nearly five years had elapsed since James Murray had been appointed editor. Twenty-seven years had passed since Richard Chenevix Trench had given his famous address in which he called for a new English dictionary. Now, in a muddy off-white cover and with its sheets half uncut, was the first part, 352 pages' worth of all the known English words from *A* to *Ant*, published by the Clarendon Press, Oxford, at a price of twelve shillings and sixpence.

Here, at last, was the first morsel of substance: part one of *A New English Dictionary on Historical Principles, Founded Mainly on the Materials Collected by The Philological Society, edited by James A. H. Murray, LL.D., Sometime President of the Philological Society, with the Assistance of Many Scholars and Men of Science.*

Murray could not help but be proud; the problems that seemed so insuperable, and that so pressed down on him, would tend to vanish whenever he held the flimsy paper-covered volume in his hand. And in a sudden sunburst of birthday-eve optimism, the editor—he would be forty-seven in less than a week—declared that he now felt confident in predicting that the final part would be published in eleven years' time.

It was in fact to take another forty-four.

But now, after all the years of waiting, the interested world could at least see the magnificent complexity of the undertaking, the detail, the filigree work, the sheer intricacies of exactitude that the editors were bent on compiling. Those in England could write and receive a copy for 12s. 6d; those in the United States received a fascicle printed in Oxford, but published by Macmillan in New York, for $3.25.

The first part's first word—once the four pages devoted to the simple letter *a* had been accounted for—was the obsolete noun *aa*, meaning "a stream" or "a watercourse." There was a quotation supporting its existence from a work of 1430, which had a reference to the still rather damp and water-girt Lincolnshire town of Saltfleetby, in which, four centuries earlier, there had been a rivulet known locally as "*le Seventown Aa.*"

The first properly current word in the fascicle was *aal*, a Bengali or Hindi name for a plant related to the madder, from which a dye could be extracted and used to color clothes. Andrew Ure's 1839 *Dictionary of Arts, Manufactures and Mines* provided the authority: "He has obtained from the aal root a pale yellow substance which he calls morindin."

And then the first properly English word—if, a linguist might quibble, there ever is such a thing. It was to be *aardvark*, the half armadillo, half anteater that lives in sub-Saharan Africa and has a sticky two-foot tongue. Three quotations are offered, the earliest from 1833.

Thus does the vast emporium of words begin to display itself, through *acatalectic* and *adhesion*, via *agnate* and *allumine*, to *animal, answer*, and, finally, to *ant*. By that last, Murray's team meant a great deal more than "simply the small social insect of the Hymenopterous order"; there is also the contraction for *ain't*, a rare prefix meaning "anti-," as with *antacid*, and more commonly the suffix derived from the French for "sometimes," and appended to make words like *tenant, val-iant, claimant,* and *pleasant.* Three hundred and fifty pages of scholarly amassment, the first pages of what would in more than four decades' time swell to no fewer than 15,487.

It was in the new Scriptorium in Oxford that Doctor Murray was to do all future work on the dictionary. He and Ada and their considerable family—six sons and five daughters—had moved there in the summer of 1884, six months after *A-Ant.* They had taken a large house on what were then the northern outskirts of the city, at 78 Banbury Road. It was called Sunnyside. The house, large and comfort-able in the manner of North Oxford, which is a sedate settling ground for the university's greater dons and lesser institutes, exists still, together with the red pillarbox that the Post Of-fice erected outside to swallow up the immense amounts of outgoing letters. Today the house is occupied by a popular anthropologist, and he has changed it little enough on the outside.

Only the Scriptorium—the Scrippy, as the Murray family knew it, which Murray's own dictionary defines as "the room in a religious house set apart for the copying of manuscripts"—has gone. Perhaps not surprisingly: No one, even in Victorian times, much liked the iron-and-corrugated-tin construction, fifteen feet by fifty, that was put up in the back garden. The next-door neighbor said it spoiled his view, and so Murray had it sunk into a three-foot-deep trench, which made it damp and cold for the staff and produced a huge bank of discarded earth that offended the neighbors even more. When it was finished, people said it looked like a tool shed, a stable, or a washhouse, and those who labored in it cursed the monkish asceticism of its construction and its irredeemably bone-chilling cold, and called it "a horrid, corrugated den."

But it was twenty feet longer than the Mill Hill Scriptorium (which does still exist, an annex to the library of what is still a costly and fashionable school), and the arrangements for filing, sorting, and then using the incoming quotation slips—which by now were flooding in at the rate of more than a thousand each day—were much improved.

There were 1,029 pigeonholes built at first (Coleridge had just 54); then banks of shelves were built as the volume and the sheer weight of slips became unmanageably large. Long and well-polished mahogany tables supported the texts selected for the word of the day or the hour, and large churchly lecterns held up the main dictionaries and reference books to which Murray and his men made constant reference. The leader himself had placed his seat and desk on a dais back in the Mill Hill days; here at Oxford there was a more democratically level floor, but Murray's stool was taller than the rest, and he presided from it still with unchallenged authority, seeing all, missing little.

He organized the workings of the Scriptorium as might an officer on a battlefield. The slips were the peculiar province of the quartermaster corps, of which Murray was quartermaster general. The packages would come in each morning, a thousand or so slips a day. One reader would check quickly to see if the quotation was full and all words were spelled properly; then a second—often one of Murray's children, each of whom was employed almost as soon as he or she was literate, paid sixpence a week for half an hour a day and rendered precociously crossword capable—would sort the contents of each bundle into the catchwords' alphabetical order. A third worker would then divide the catchwords into their various recognized parts of speech—*bell* as noun, *bell* as adjective, *bell* as verb, for instance—and then a fourth employee would see that the quotations assembled for each were arranged chronologically.

Then a subeditor, one of the more exalted members of the team, would subdivide the meanings of each word into the various shades it had enjoyed over its lifetime; also at this point (if he had not done so earlier) he would make a first stab at writing that most crucial feature of most dictionaries—the definition.

Defining words properly is a fine and peculiar craft. There are rules—a word (to take a noun as an example) must first be defined according to the class of things to which it belongs (mammal, quadruped), and then differentiated from other members of that class (bovine, female). There must be no words in the definition that are more complicated or less likely to be known than the word being defined. The definition must say what something is, and not what it is not. If there is a range of meanings of any one word—*cow* having a broad range of meanings, *cower* having essentially only one—then they must be stated. And all the words in the definition must be found elsewhere in the dictionary—a reader must never happen upon a word in the dictionary that he or she cannot discover elsewhere in it. If the definer contrives to follow all these rules, stirs into the mix an ever-pressing need for concision and elegance—and if he or she is true to the task, a proper definition will probably result.

By now the words from the envelope of quotations would have been assembled into the smallest of subgroups, each with a stated meaning and a definition—either just written by a junior, or written some time before when the word was in a half-completed state. It simply remained now to divide these subgroups chronologically, so as to demonstrate—with the army of quotations—just how the shades of meaning of the catchword had altered and evolved over its lifespan.

Once this was done, Murray would take the collections of slips for each of the subgroups for any distinct and defined target word and arrange or rearrange or further subdivide them as he saw fit. He would write and insert the word's etymology (which Oxford, despite the existence of its own etymological dictionary, did in the end see fit to allow Murray to include) and its pronunciation—a tricky decision, and one likely to provoke, as it has, ceaseless controversy—and then make a final selection of the very best quotations. Ideally there should be at least one sentence from the literature for each century in which the word was used—unless it was a very fast-changing word that needed more quotations to suggest the speed of its new shadings.

Finally, with that all squared away, Murray would write the concise, scholarly, accurate, and lovingly elegant definition for which the Dictionary is well known—and send the finished columns over to the press. It would be set in a Clarendon or an Old Style typeface (or in Greek or other foreign or Old English or Anglo-Saxon face when needed), and returned to the Scriptorium, printed in galley. It was ready to be set onto a page, and the page made into a form for placing on the great letterpress engines in the stone printing works down in the back of Walton Street.

Murray was no whiner, but his letters tell a great deal about the difficulty of the task he had set himself—and that the publishers, who wanted to see a return on their investment, in turn had set him. The expressed hope was that two parts—six hundred pages of finished dictionary—might be published each year. Murray himself tried gallantly to complete work on thirty-three words every day—and yet "often a single word, like *Approve* . . . takes ¾ of a day itself."

Murray spoke of the trials of the work in his presidential address to the Philological Society, and a subsequent *Athenaeum* article in March 1884—an article that led to his first real contact with William Minor. He referred to the difficulty "of pushing our way experimentally through an untrodden forest where no white man's ax has been before us."

> Only those who have made the experiment know the bewilderment with which editor or sub-editor, after he has apportioned the quotations for such a word as above . . . among 20, 30 or 40 groups, and furnished each of these with a provisional definition, spreads them out on a table or on the floor where he can obtain a general survey of the whole, and spends hour after hour in shifting them about like pieces on

a chess-board, striving to find in the fragmentary evidence of an incomplete historical record, such a sequence of meanings as may form a logical chain of development. Sometimes the quest seems hopeless; recently, for example, the word *art* utterly baffled me for several days: something had to be done with it: something was done and put in type; but the renewed consideration of it in print, with the greater facility of reading and comparison which this afforded, led to the entire pulling to pieces and reconstruction of the edifice, extending to several columns of type.

It was at about this time, when Murray was so very vexed over *art*, that one of his subeditors—or perhaps it was Murray himself—wrote the first official request to Broadmoor. They wanted Doctor Minor to find out if he had earmarked any quotations for *art* that suggested other meanings, or which came from earlier dates, than had been assembled so far. Sixteen distinct shades of meaning had been uncovered for the noun: Perhaps Minor had some more, or some further illumination of the word. If so, then he—and anyone else, for that matter—should kindly send them back to Oxford, posthaste.

Eighteen letters duly came in about the word from a variety of readers who had seen the article. One of the replies, undeniably the most fruitful, came from Broadmoor.

In comparison with all other readers, who had offered merely one sentence or two, the unsung Doctor Minor had enclosed no fewer than twenty-seven. He struck his subeditors in Oxford as not only a meticulous man; he was also very prolific, and able to tap deep into wells of knowledge and research. The dictionary team had made a rare find.

It has to be said that most of Minor's quotations for this particular word came from a somewhat obvious source: Sir Joshua Reynolds's famous *Discourses*, written in 1769, the year after he became president of the Royal Academy. But they were of inestimable value to the dictionary makers— and as proof, there today, standing as a mute memorial to the beginnings of his work, is the first known quotation that William Chester Minor had placed in the finished book.

It is the second quotation under the sense "*The Arts*," and it reads simply: "1769 Reynolds, Sir J. *Disc.* I Wks. 1870 306 There is a general desire among our Nobility to be distinguished as lovers and judges of the Arts."

Unwittingly, Sir Joshua's words were to provide the starting point for a relationship between Doctor Murray and Doctor Minor that would combine sublime scholarship, fierce tragedy, Victorian reserve, deep gratitude, mutual respect, and a slowly growing amity that could even, in the loosest sense, be termed friendship. Whatever it was called, it was a link that would last the two men until death finally separated them thirty years later. The work Doctor Minor did for the dictionary, and which began with Reynold's *Discourses*, continued for the next two decades; but some stronger bond than a simple love of words had also been forged, and it was one that kept these two so different elderly men intimately connected for half as long again.

It was to be seven years before they met, however. During that time Minor began to send out his quotations at a prodigious rate—at times many more than a hundred new slips every week, as many as twenty a day, all in a neat, firm hand. He would write to Murray—always rather formally, straying only rarely into matters that were not within his self-appointed purview.

The first correspondence that survives, from October 1886, was largely about agricultural matters. Perhaps the doctor, taking a break from his work at the table, had stood up to stretch and had gazed wistfully from his cell window down at the farm laborers in the valley below, watching them stacking the late autumn sheaves and drinking warm cider under the oaks. He refers in his letter to a book he is reading, called *The Country Farme*, by Gervase Markham, published in 1616, and to occurrences of the verb *bell*—as when the ripening hops swell out in bell shapes in late August. *Blight*, too, catches his attention, as well as *blast*, and then *heckling*, which on farms once meant the process of separating the individual stems of the flax plant from each other, and only later became used (often in a political context) in the sense of catechizing someone, making his or her arguments stand up to severe scrutiny, as a flax plant might stand when divided for the scutcher.

He likes the word *buckwheat* too—and its French translation *blé noir*—and finds such niceties as "ointment of buckwheat." He clearly revels in his work: One can almost feel him squirming with something akin to teenage excitement as he offers: "I could give you more if you wanted," and as a teasing bonus throws in a small temptation on the thoroughly amusing word *horsebread*. He signs off, seeming to will a response from the great man on the great outside: "I trust same may be useful to you—Very truly yours, W. C. Minor, Broadmoor. Crowthorne. Berks."

The tone of this and other such letters as survive seems halfway between the obsequious and the detached: dignified and controlled on the one hand, and leavened with Uriah Heep–like toadying on the other. Minor wants desperately to know that he is being helpful. He wants to feel involved. He wants, but knows he can never demand, that praise be showered on him. He wants respectability, and he wants those in the asylum to know that he is special, different from others in their cells.

Though he has no idea at all of his correspondent's character or circumstances—thinking him still a practicing medical man of literary tastes with a good deal of leisure—Murray seems to recognize something of his pleading tone. He notices, for instance, the curious way Minor seems to prefer to work on those words that are current—like *art* first and then *blast* and *buckwheat*—and that are in the process of being placed into the succession of pages, parts, and volumes of the moment. Murray notes in a letter to a colleague that Minor clearly very much wants to stay up to date—that unlike most other readers he has no interest in working on words that are destined for volumes and letters to be published years and decades hence. The editor writes later that he feels Minor clearly wants to be able *to feel involved*, to enjoy the impression that he, Minor, is somehow a part of the team, doing things in tandem with the scribes up at the Scriptorium.

Minor was none too far from Oxford, after all—perhaps he felt as though he were at a detached college, like St. Catherine's Society or Mansfield Hall, and that his cells—or what James Murray still thought of as his comfortable, book-lined brown study—were just a rurally detached edition of the Scriptorium, a den of scholarly creation and lexical detective work. Had anyone chosen to ponder further, he or she might have wondered at the strange symmetry of the two men's settings—pinioned as each was among great stacks of books, single-mindedly devoted to learning of the most recondite kind, each man's only outlet his correspondence, in great daily storms of paper and floods of ink.

Except there was a difference: William Minor remained profoundly and irreversibly mad.

The Broadmoor attendants had noticed some improvement in the very early 1880s, when he first replied to the appeal from Mill Hill. But as the years went on, and as Minor passed dejected and alone through the milestone of his fiftieth birthday in June 1884—his elderly stepmother having visited him the month before, on her way home to the United States from Ceylon, where she had stayed since her husband's death—so the old ills returned, reinvigorated, reinforced.

"Dear Dr. Orange," he writes to the Broadmoor superintendent at the beginning of the next September. "The defacement of my books still goes on. It is simply certain that someone besides myself has access to them, and abuses it."

His handwriting is shaky, uncertain. He heard his cell door opening at 3 A.M. the night before, he says, and goes on, raving, "The sound of that door, as you may verify, since the alteration, is unmistakable; and you could be as morally sure of its closure by the sound, as of anything you do not really see." If he has no other remedy, he warns, "I shall have to send my books back to London, and have them sold." Thankfully this small tantrum was short-lived. Had it continued or worsened, the dictionary might have lost one of its closest and most valuable friends.

A month later a new obsession grips him:

> Dear Dr. Orange—Let me mention one fact that falls in with my hypothesis. So many fires have occurred in the U.S. originating quite inexplicably in the interspace of ceiling and floor that, I learn now, Insurance Companies refuse to ensure large buildings—mills, factories—which have the usual hollow spacing under the floor. They insist upon solid floors. All this has come to notice within ten years; but no-one suggests any explanation.

Except Doctor Minor, that is. Fiends have been creeping about in the interstices between floors and ceilings and have wrought mischief and committed crimes—not least in Broadmoor, where they hide and crawl out at night, to abuse the poor doctor nightly, mark his books, steal his flute, and torture him cruelly. The hospital, he says, must have solid floors built in: otherwise, no fire insurance, and a host of nightly misdeeds.

The daily reports flow in a kind of seamless syrup of insanity. Four cakes stolen; his flute gone; his books all marked; he himself frog-marched up and down the corridor by Attendants James and Annett. A spare key used at night to allow villagers into his rooms to abuse him and his possessions. Doctor Minor, in his drawers and shirt, stockings and slippers, complaining that small pieces of wood were forced into his lock, that electricity was used on his body, that a *"murderous lot"* had beaten him during the night and had left a savage pain all along his left side. Scoundrels came to his room. Attendant Coles came at 6 A.M. and *"used my body"*—"It is *a very dirty business,"* he screamed one morning, standing now only in his drawers, *"that a fellow cannot sleep without Coles coming in like that."* Again as before: *"He made a pimp of me!"*

And yet as came the madness, so came the words. Many of those that fascinated him were Anglo-Indian, reflecting his birthplace: There were *bhang, brinjal, catamaran, cholera, chunnam,* and *cutcherry.* He liked *brick-tea.* By the time of the middle 1890s he became very active working on the letter *D,* and though there are some Hindustani words like *dubash, dubba,* and *dhobi,* he was interested also in what were regarded as the core words of the dictionary—and contributions of quotations are in the Oxford archives for such words as *delicately, directly, dirt, disquiet, drink, duty,* and *dye.* He was able more often than not to supply the quotation for the first use of a word—always an occasion for celebration. For the use of the word *dirt* meaning "earth," he quotes from John Fryer's *New Account of East Indies and Persia,* published in 1698. For one meaning of *magnificence,* for one of *model,* for *reminiscence,* and for *spalt,* a foolish person, the first work by du Boscq also provided ideal material.

The dictionary staff at Oxford noticed only one small and strange rhythm to Minor's frantic pace: that in the high summertime rather fewer packages would come. Perhaps, they speculated innocently, Doctor Minor liked to spend the warm days outside, away from his books—a reasonable explanation indeed. But when the autumn came around again, and the evening began to darken, so he began working ceaselessly again, replying to every request, asking repeatedly and anxiously about the progress of the work, and inundating the team with ever more packages of slips—more quotations, even, than were needed.

"One could wish that Dr. Minor had made about half the number of references," wrote Murray to another editor, overwhelmed, "but indeed one never really knows what words will come of use till one comes to deal with the word lexicographically."

Because his method of working was very different from everyone else's, it is more difficult to make a quantitative comparison, to set the numerical achievement of his work against that of the other great contributors. Perhaps at the end of the project he had actually sent in no more than ten thousand slips, which sounds a fairly modest number. But as virtually all of them proved to be useful, and because every one of them was wanted, and had been ordered, so his achievement as a contributor more than equals the effort achieved by some others in sending ten thousand slips *a year*.

The Oxford team was indeed grateful. The preface to the first completed volume, volume 1, A-B, when finished in 1888—a full nine years after the project was begun—contains a one-line mention. It might as well have been a page of fulsome thanks, and it made their contributor supremely proud, not least because it was, by happenstance, discreet enough to offer no hint to others of his strange situation. It said simply and elegantly: "Dr. W. C. Minor of Crowthorne."

Grateful though they might have been, the Oxford team was also becoming, as time went on, very, very puzzled. And Murray was more puzzled than all of them.

Who exactly was this brilliant, strange, exacting man? they asked one another. Murray attempted, fruitlessly, to inquire. Crowthorne was less than forty miles from Oxford, an hour by the Great Western Railway via Reading. How was it that Minor, so distinguished and energetic a man, and so much a neighbor, was never to be seen? How could there be a man of such lexicographical skills, who had so much leisure and energy and lived so very close, and who yet never seemed to want to see the temple to which he sent so many thousands of offerings? Where was the man's curiosity? What was his pleasure? Was he somehow unwell, disabled, frightened? Could it be that he felt intimidated by the company of great Oxford men like these?

The answer to the deepening mystery came about in a curious manner. It was delivered to Doctor Murray by a passing scholar-librarian, who stopped by at the Scriptorium in 1889 to talk about more serious matters. In the course of a talk that ranged across the entire spectrum of lexicography, he made a chance reference to the Crowthorne doctor.

How kind the good James Murray had evidently been to him, remarked the scholar. "How good you have been to our poor Dr. Minor."

There was a startling pause, and the subeditors and secretaries in the Scriptorium who had overheard the conversation suddenly stopped in their tracks. As one, they looked up, toward where their leader and his visitor were sitting.

"*Poor* Dr. Minor?" asked Murray, as perplexed as any one of those who were now keenly listening. "*What can you possibly mean?*"

9

The Meeting of Minds

‖ **Dénouement** (denū·maṅ). [F. *dénouement*, *dénoûment*, formerly *desnouement*, f. *dénouer*, *desnouer*, in OF. *desnoer* to untie = Pr. *denozar*, It. *disnodare*, a Romanic formation from L. *dis-* + *nodāre* to knot, *nodus* knot.]

Unravelling; *spec.* the final unravelling of the complications of a plot in a drama, novel, etc.; the catastrophe; *transf.* the final solution or issue of a complication, difficulty, or mystery.

Modern literary myth maintains, even today, that the strangest puzzle surrounding William Chester Minor's career was this: Just why did he not attend the great dictionary dinner—a dinner to which he was invited—held in Oxford on the glittering evening of Tuesday, October 12, 1897?

It was Queen Victoria's Jubilee Year, and those who were connected with the *OED* project were in more than a mood

for a party. The dictionary was at long last going well. The fal-
tering progress of the early years was now accelerating—the
fascicle *Anta-Battening* had been published in 1885, *Battentlie-
Bozzom* in 1887, *Bra-Byzen* in 1888. A new spirit of efficiency
had settled on the Scriptorium. And as crowning glory Queen
Victoria had in 1896 "graciously agreed," as the court liked
to say, that the just-completed volume 3—embracing the
entirety of the infuriating letter *C* (which the lexicographers
found unusually filled with ambiguities and complexities,
not least because of its frequent overlaps with the letters *G, K,*
and *S*)—should be dedicated to her.

An aura of majestic permanence had all of a sudden in-
vested the dictionary. There was no doubt now that it would
eventually be completed—for since it had been royally approved, who could ever brook its cancellation? With that
happy realization, and with the queen having done her part,
so Oxford, in high mood for celebration, decided it could
follow suit. James Murray deserved to be given honors and
thanks—and who more appropriate than the great man's adopted university to bestow them?

The university's new vice-chancellor decided that a big
dinner—"slap-up," to employ a phrase that the dictionary
was to quote from 1823—should be held in Murray's honor.
It would be staged in the huge hall at the Queen's College,
where by old tradition a scholar with a silver trumpet sounds
a fanfare to summon guests in to dine. It would celebrate
what *The Times*, on the day of the dinner, proclaimed to be
"the greatest effort probably which any university, it may be
any printing press, has taken in hand since the invention of

printing. . . . It will not be the least of the glories of the University of Oxford to have completed this gigantic task." The evening would be a memorable Oxford event.

As indeed it was. The long tables were splendidly decorated with flowers and with all the best silverware and crystal that Queen's could roust from its cellars. The menu was forthright and English—clear turtle soup, turbot with lobster sauce, haunch of mutton, roast partridges, Queen Mab pudding, and strawberry ice. But like the dictionary itself, it was also flavored generously, but not too generously, with Gallicisms: "sweet-breads after the mode of Villeroi, grenadines of veal, ramequins." The wines were plentiful and excellent: an 1858 amontillado sherry, an 1882 Adriatic maraschino liqueur, an aged Château d'Yquem, and champagne by Pfungst, 1889. The guests wore white tie, academic robes, medals. During the speeches—and after a "loyal toast" in which the graciousness of her majesty was duly noted, and her six decades on the throne proudly congratulated, they smoked cigars.

They must have smoked long and well. There were no fewer than fourteen speeches—James Murray on the entire history of dictionary making, the head of the Oxford University Press on his belief that the project was a great duty to the nation, and the egregious Henry Furnivall, as lively and amusing as ever, taking time from recruiting buxom Amazons from the local ABC teahouse to come a-rowing with him, to speak on what he saw as Oxford's heartless attitude toward the admission of women.

Among the guests could be counted all the great and the good of the academic land. The editors of the dictionary, the

Delegates of the press, the printers, members of the Philological Society, and, not least, some of the most assiduous and energetic of the volunteer readers.

There was Mr. F. T. Elworthy of Wellington; Miss J. E. A. Brown of Further Barton, near Cirencester; the Rev. W. E. Smith of Putney; Lord Aldenham (better known by friends of the dictionary as Mr. H. Huck Gibbs); Mr. Russell Martineau; Monsieur F. J. Amours; and for the later parts of D, the Misses Edith and E. Perronet Thompson, both of Reigate. The list was long: but so sonorous were the names and so evidently awesome their achievements, the diners, well into their port and cognac by now, heard them out in a silence that was easy to confuse with rapture.

As it happens, the most fulsome remarks made about the volunteers that night relate to two men who had much in common: Both were Americans, both spent time in India, both were soldiers, both were mad, and though both had been invited, neither one came to the Oxford dinner.

The first was Dr. Fitzedward Hall, who came from Troy, New York. His was a bizarre story. Just as he was about to enter Harvard in 1848, his family demanded that he set off for Calcutta to track down an errant brother. His ship was wrecked in the Bay of Bengal; he survived and became fascinated by Sanskrit, studying it to the point where he was eventually offered the chair in Sanskrit at Government College in Varanasi, then called Benares, the holiest city in the Ganges Valley. He fought for the British side during the Sepoy Mutiny in 1857, as a rifleman; then left India in 1860 and became Sanskrit professor at King's College, London, and librarian at the India Office.

And then, quite precipitously, his life fell terribly apart. No one is sure why, except that he had a furious dispute with a fellow Sanskrit scholar from Austria named Theodor Goldstücker. It was a dispute of such gravity—linguists and philologists were known to be mercurial and hold eternal grudges—that it caused Hall to quit the India Office, have himself summarily suspended from the Philological Society, and leave London for a small village in Suffolk.

People said he was a drunkard, a foreign spy, hopelessly immoral, and an academic phony. He in turn accused all Britons of turning on him, ruining his life, driving away his wife, and displaying only a "fiendish hatred" of Americans. He turned the key in the lock of his cottage in Marlesford, and—except for the occasional steamer voyage back home to New York—lived the life of a near-total country recluse.

And yet he wrote every single day to James Murray at Oxford—a correspondence that continued for twenty years. The two men never met—but over the years Hall without complaint compiled slips, answered queries, offered advice, and remained the staunchest ally of the dictionary during its bleakest days. Small wonder that Doctor Murray wrote in the great preface: "[A]bove all we have to record the inestimable collaboration of Dr. Fitzedward Hall, whose voluntary labours have completed the literary and documentary history of numberless words, senses and idioms, and whose contributions are to be found on every page."

Those at the dinner knew why he had not come: They knew that he was a hermit, that he was difficult. But no one knew—or so the story has long had it—exactly why the man next mentioned had not turned up. Murray, in writing the celebrated preface, had been almost equally generous in his praise: "also the unflagging services of Dr. W. C. Minor, which have week by week supplied additional quotations for the words actually preparing for press." "Second only to the contributions of Dr. Fitzedward Hall," Murray was to write a little later, "in enhancing our illustration of the literary history of individual words, phrases and constructions, have been those of Dr. W. C. Minor, received week by week."

But where, wondered the gathered assembly, *was* Doctor Minor? He was living at Crowthorne, only sixty minutes away by the green-and-gold steam trains of the Great Western. He was not notorious as an ill-tempered misanthrope, like Doctor Hall. His letters had always been noted for their polite solicitousness. So why could he not have had the courtesy to come? To some who dined at Queen's on that glorious autumn evening, Minor's absence must have seemed a melancholy footnote to an otherwise glorious literary moment.

The received wisdom has it that Doctor Murray was perplexed, even vaguely irritated. It is said that he vowed, out of all his lexicographic knowledge, to take a leaf from Francis Bacon, who in 1624 had written in English the axiom from the collection of the Prophet's sayings known as the *hadith*, to the effect that "If the mountain will not come to Mahomet, then Mahomet must go to the mountain."

It is said that he promptly wrote to Doctor Minor, his letter supposedly reading as follows:

> You and I have now known each other through correspondence for fully seventeen years, and it is a sad fact that we have never met. Perhaps it has never proved convenient for you to travel; maybe it has been too expensive; but while it is difficult indeed for me to leave the work of the Scriptorium even for one day, I have long wanted to meet you, and may I perhaps suggest that I come to visit you. If this is convenient, perhaps you might suggest a day and a train, and if convenient for me I will telegraph the time of my expected arrival.

Doctor Minor supposedly wrote back promptly, saying that he would of course be delighted to receive the editor, that he was so sorry that physical circumstances—he did not elaborate—had hitherto made it impossible for him to come up to Oxford, and suggested a number of trains from those listed in the *Bradshaw*. Murray duly selected a November Wednesday, and a train that, with a change in Reading, was due into the Wellington College railway station shortly after lunch.

He telegraphed the details to Crowthorne, wheeled out his faithful black Humber tricycle, and, with his white beard blowing over his shoulder in the chilly breeze, set out down the Banbury Road, past the Randolph Hotel, the Ashmolean

Museum, and Worcester College, and to the Up, or London-bound, platform of Oxford Station.

The journey took just a little over an hour. He was pleasantly surprised, on arriving at Crowthorne, to find a brougham and a liveried coachman waiting for him. His long-held assumption that Minor must be a leisured man of letters was reinforced: Perhaps, he thought to himself, he was even a man of means.

The horses clip-clopped through the fog-damp lanes. The magnificent pile of Wellington School lay neatly in the distance, a respectable distance from Crowthorne village itself, which was no more than a cluster of cottages, the piles of lawn leaves smoldering behind them. It was a pretty little place, quiet, well wooded, and rather self-contained.

After a couple of miles the coachman swung the horses into a poplar-lined driveway that climbed a long, low hill. The cottages thinned out and were replaced by a number of small red-brick houses of a rather more severe look. Then the horses stopped before an imposing front gate, a pair of towers with a great black-faced clock between, and green-painted doors that were being opened by a servant. The editor was perhaps vaguely excited: This must have seemed to him a grand country house in which he was being exceedingly well received, as though expected for a sumptuous afternoon tea, or like someone arriving at Kedleston for luncheon with Lord Curzon.

James Murray removed his cap and unbuttoned the Inverness tweed cape that had protected him from the cold. The servant said nothing, but ushered him inside and up a flight of marble stairs. He was swept into a large room with a glowing coal fire and a wall covered with portraits of gaunt-looking men. There was a large director's desk, and behind it, a portly man of obvious importance. The servant backed out and closed the door.

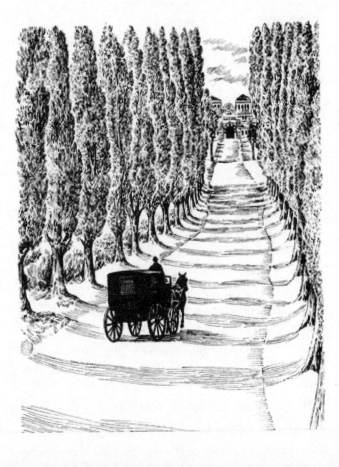

Murray advanced toward the great man, who rose. Murray bowed stiffly and extended his hand.

"I, Sir, am Dr. James Murray of the London Philological Society," he said in his finely modulated Scottish voice, "and editor of the *Oxford English Dictionary*.

"And you sir, must be Dr. William Minor. At long last. I am most deeply honoured to meet you."

There was a pause. Then the other man replied:

"I regret not, sir. I cannot lay claim to that distinction. I am the Superintendent of the Broadmoor Criminal Lunatic Asylum. Dr. Minor is an American, and he is one of our longest-staying inmates. He committed a murder. He is quite insane."

Doctor Murray, as the story then continues, was in turn astonished, amazed, and yet filled with sympathetic interest. "He begged to be taken to Doctor Minor, and the meeting between the two men of learning who had corresponded for so long and who now met in such strange circumstances was an extremely impressive one."

The story of this first meeting is, however, no more than an amusing and romantic fiction. It was created by an American journalist named Hayden Church, who lived in London for most of the first half of this century. It first appeared in England in the *Strand* magazine in September 1915, and then again, revised and amplified, in the same journal six months later.

In fact Church had already tried it out on an American audience, writing anonymously for the *Sunday Star* in Washington, D.C., in July 1915. The story was splendidly sensationalized, with the kind of lurid, multilayered headline that has sadly gone almost out of fashion.

AMERICAN MURDERER HELPED WRITE OXFORD DICTIONARY, read the first, extending over all eight columns of the page. MYSTERIOUS CONTRIBUTOR TO AN ENGLISH DICTIONARY PROVED TO BE A RICH AMERICAN SURGEON CONFINED IN BROADMOOR CRIMINAL LUNATIC ASYLUM FOR A MURDER COMMITTED WHILE HE WAS IN A DERANGED CONDITION—HOW SIR JAMES MURRAY, EDITOR OF THE DICTIONARY, WHO SET OUT, AS HE THOUGHT, TO VISIT THE HOME OF A FELLOW SAVANT, FOUND HIMSELF AT THE ASYLUM AND HEARD THE EXTRAORDINARY TALE, WHICH BEGINS DURING THE AMERICAN CIVIL WAR WHEN THE PRINCIPAL WAS A SURGEON IN THE NORTHERN ARMY—CONTRIBUTOR WEALTHY AND NOW LIVING IN AMERICA, SAYS HIS FRIEND.

The breathless headline told of an even more exhausting story—but one made more than faintly ludicrous by its author's inability or unwillingness to name Minor. In every reference he is called simply Doctor Blank, as in "And you sir, must be Dr. Blank. I am most honoured to meet you."

The story nonetheless went down well with its American audience, which had been given hints and snippets in the years before—the arrest of one of their officers for murder in London not having passed unnoticed at the time, his imprisonment receiving occasional dustings-off as new correspondents and new diplomats found their way to the English capital. But the revelation of his work for the dictionary was new, and in this regard Hayden Church had a good, old-fashioned scoop. The wires picked the story up; it appeared in papers around the world, and as far away as Tientsin, China.

But in London it did not go down so well. Henry Bradley, who by this time had taken over from Murray as editor in chief of what was now formally known as the *Oxford English Dictionary*, took exception to the *Strand* article. He wrote an angry letter to the *Daily Telegraph*, complaining of "several misstatements of fact," and that "the story of Dr. Murray's first interview with Dr. Minor is, so far as its most romantic features are concerned, a fiction."

Hayden Church dashed off a spirited reply to Bradley, which the *Telegraph*, naturally liking a fight, happily published. It contains vague rebuttals, citing only "a host of correspondents, some of them of great eminence"—but none of whom are named—who had confirmed the major aspects of the story. It pleads, limply, that "I have the best of reasons for believing the account of the meeting between Minor and Murray to be accurate."

The oddest part of Church's reply, however, is its enigmatic postscript. "I have just been in communication with one of the most distinguished literary men in England, who . . . pointed out that *there did not appear in my article what he personally considered the most striking feature of all in the American's history* [emphasis added]."

Strictly true or not, Hayden Church's account of the first meeting turned out to be simply far too good to ignore. It enthralled all England, people said. It took their mind off

World War I—1915, after all, was the year of Ypres, of Gallip-
oli, of the sinking of the *Lusitania*, and people were no doubt
content to have such a saga as a diversion from the grim real-
ities of the fighting. "No romance," said the *Pall Mall Gazette*,
"is equal to this wonderful story, of scholarship in a padded
cell."

Virtually all subsequent references to the saga of Oxford dictionary making retell Church's story, to a greater or
lesser degree. In her justly celebrated biography (1977) of her
grandfather, Miss K. M. Elisabeth Murray retells Church's
version of events almost without question, as does Jonathon
Green in a more general book on the history of lexicography,
published in 1996. Only Elizabeth Knowles, an Oxford University Press editor who became intrigued by the story in the
early 1990s, takes a cooler and more detached view: Still,
she is clearly perplexed that no definitive account of the first
meeting can be found. The patina applied by decades of good
use has made the legend pleasingly credible.

The truth, however, turns out to be only marginally less
romantic. It surfaces in a letter Murray wrote in 1902 to a distinguished friend, Dr. Francis Brown, in Boston, and which
turned up in a wooden box in the attic of one of William Minor's very few living relations, a retired businessman living
in Riverside, Connecticut. The letter appears to be the full
and complete original, although it was the exhausting habit
of many letter writers of the time to prepare a fair copy of all
their outgoing mail, and in so doing occasionally to edit and
elide some passages.

*   *   *

His first contact with Minor, writes Doctor Murray, came
very soon after the beginning of his work in the dictionary—
probably 1880 or even 1881. "He proved to be a very good
reader, who wrote to me often," and, as has already been mentioned, Murray thought only that he must be a retired medical man with plenty of time on his hands:

> By accident, my attention was called to the fact
> that his address, *Broadmoor, Crowthorne*, Berk-
> shire, was that of a large lunatic asylum. I assumed
> that (perhaps) he was the medical officer of that
> institution.
>
> But our correspondence was of course entirely lim-
> ited to the Dictionary and its materials, and the only
> feeling I had towards him was that of gratitude for his
> immense help, with some surprise at the rare and ex-
> pensive old books that he evidently had access to.
>
> This continued for years until one day, between
> 1887 and 1890, the late Mr. Justin Winsor, Librarian
> of Harvard College, was sitting chatting in my Scrip-
> torium and among other things remarked "you have
> given great pleasure to Americans by speaking as you
> do in your Preface of poor Dr. Minor. This is a very
> painful case."
>
> "Indeed," I said with astonishment, "in what way?"
>
> Mr. W. was equally astonished to find that in all
> these years I had corresponded with Dr. Minor I had

never learned nor suspected anything about him; and he then thrilled me with his story.

The great librarian—for Justin Winsor remains one of the grandest figures in all of nineteenth-century American librarianship, and a formidable historian to boot—then told the story, which Murray then retold to his friend in Boston. Some of the facts are wrong, as facts tend to be when related over a period of years—Murray says that Minor went to Harvard (while in fact he went to Yale), and repeats the probably apocryphal story that he was driven mad by having to witness the execution of two men after a court-martial. He goes on to say that the shooting happened in the Strand—then, unlike now, one of London's more fashionable streets—rather than in the grim purlieus of the Lambeth waterside. But essentially the story is relayed correctly, after which Murray resumes his own narrative.

I was of course deeply affected by the story; but as Dr. Minor had never in the least alluded to himself or his position, all I could do was to write to him more respectfully and kindly than before, so as to show no notice of this disclosure, which I feared might make some change in our relations.

A few years ago an American citizen who called on me told me he had been to see Dr. Minor and said he found him rather low and out of spirits, and urged me to go to see him. I said I shrank from that, because I had no reason to suppose that Dr. Minor thought I knew anything about him personally.

He said: "Yes, he does. He has no doubt that you know all about him, and it really would be a kindness if you would go and see him."

I then wrote to Dr. Minor telling him that, and that Mr. (I forget the name) who had recently visited him had told me that a visit from me would be welcome. I also wrote to Dr. Nicholson, the then Governor, who warmly invited me—and when I went, drove me from and to the Railway Station and invited me to lunch, at which he also had Dr. Minor, who I found was a great favorite with his children.

I sat with Dr. Minor in his room or cell many hours altogether before and after lunch, and found him, as far as I could see, as sane as myself, a much cultivated and scholarly man, with many artistic tastes, and of fine Christian character, quite resigned to his sad lot, and grieved only on account of the restriction it imposed on his usefulness.

I learned (from the Governor, I think) that he has always given a large part of his income to support the widow of the man whose death he so sadly caused, and that she regularly visits him.

Dr. Nicholson had a great opinion of him, gave him many privileges and regularly took distinguished visitors up to his room or cell, to see him and his books. But his successor the present governor has not shown such special sympathy.

The meeting took place in January 1891—six years earlier than is favored by the romantics who repeat the dictionary dinner story. Murray had written to Nicholson asking for permission, and in the letter we can almost feel his childlike, knee-squeezing anticipation of the event.

> It will give me great satisfaction to make the acquaintance of Dr. Minor, to whom the Dictionary owes so much, as well as yourself who have been so kind to him. I shall probably come by the train you name (the 12 from Reading) but have not had time to look up the time-table, or rather to ask my wife to do so; for in such matters I deliver myself automatically into her hands, and she tells me, "Your train starts so and so, and you will go by such a train, and I will come into the Scriptorium and fetch you to get ready five minutes before." I thankfully comply, and do my work until the "five minutes before" arrives.

It is now abundantly clear that the two men knew each other personally, and saw each other regularly, for almost twenty years from that date. The first encounter over lunch was to begin a long and firm friendship, based both on a wary mutual respect, and, more particularly, on their passionate and keenly shared love for words.

For both men, the first sight of the other must have been peculiar indeed, for they were uncannily similar in appearance. Both were tall, thin, and bald. Both had deeply hooded

blue eyes, neither using spectacles (though Minor was profoundly myopic). Doctor Minor's nose looks a little hooked,
Doctor Murray's finer and more aquiline. Minor has an air
of avuncular kindliness; Murray much the same, but with a
trace of the severity that might well distinguish a lowland
Scot from a Connecticut Yankee.

But what was most obviously similar about the men were
their beards—in both cases white, long, and nicely swallow-
tailed—with thick moustaches, sideburns, and ample bug-
gers' grips. Both looked like popular illustrations of Father
Time; boys in Oxford would see Murray tricycling by and
call out, "Father Christmas!" at him.

True, Doctor Minor's had a more ragged and unkempt
look about it, doubtless because the arrangements for cutting
and washing inside Broadmoor were rather less sophisticated
than in the outside world. Murray's beard, on the other hand,
was fine and well-combed and shampooed, and looked as
though no particle of food had ever been allowed to rest there.
Minor's was the more homely, while Murray's was more of
a fashion statement. But both were magnificently fecund arrangements. When the beards were added to the other collections of the pair's individual attributes, each must have
imagined, for a second, that he was stepping toward himself
in a looking-glass, rather than meeting a stranger.

The two men met dozens of times in the next several
years. By all accounts they liked each other—a liking subject only to Doctor Minor's moods, to which Murray became
over the years fully sensitive. He often had the foresight to
telegraph Nicholson, to ask how the patient was; if low and

angry, he would remain at Oxford; if low and likely to be comforted, he would board the train.

When the weather was poor the men would sit together in Minor's room—a small and practically furnished cell not too dissimilar from a typical Oxford student's room, and just like the room Murray was to be given at Balliol, once he was made an honorary fellow. It was lined with bookshelves, all of which were open except for one glass-fronted case that held the rarest of the sixteenth- and seventeenth-century works from which much of the *OED* work was being done. The fireplace crackled merrily. Tea and Dundee cake were brought in by a fellow inmate whom Minor had hired to work for him— one of the many privileges Nicholson, like Orange before him, accorded his distinguished inmate.

There was a whole raft of other perks besides. He was able to order books at will from various antiquarian dealers in London, New York, and Boston. He was able to write uncensored letters to whomever he chose. He was able to have visitors more or less at will—and told Murray with some pride that Eliza Merrett, the widow of the man he murdered, would come to his rooms quite frequently. She was not an unattractive woman, he said, though it was thought that she drank rather too much for comfort.

He subscribed to magazines, which he and Murray would read to each other: The *Spectator* was one of his favorites, and *Outlook*, which was mailed to him by his relations in Connecticut. He took the *Athenaeum*, as well as the splendidly arcane Oxford publication *Notes & Queries*, which even today makes puzzling inquiries of the world's literary community, about unsolved mysteries of the bookish world. The *OED* used to publish its word desiderata there; until Murray began visiting Crowthorne, this was Minor's principal means of finding out which particular words the *OED* staff were working on.

Although the men talked principally about words—most often about a specific word, but sometimes about more general lexical problems of dialect and the nuances of pronunciation—they did, it is certain, discuss in a general sense the nature of the doctor's illness. Murray could not help noticing, for instance, that Minor's cell floor had been covered with a sheet of zinc—"to prevent men coming in through the timbers at night"—and that he kept a bowl of water beside the door of whichever room he was in—"because the evil spirits will not dare to cross water to get to me."

Murray was aware, too, of the doctor's fears that he would be transported from his room at night and made to perform "deeds of the wildest excess" in "dens of infamy" before being returned to his cell by dawn. Once airplanes were invented—and Minor, being American, kept keenly up to date with all that happened in the years after the Wright Brothers first flew at Kitty Hawk—he incorporated them into his delusions. Men would then break into his rooms, place him in a flying machine, and take him to brothels in Constantinople, where he would be forced to perform acts of terrible lewdness with cheap women and small girls. Murray winced as he heard these tales, but held his tongue. It was not his place to regard the old man with anything other than sad affection; and besides, his work for the dictionary continued apace.

When the weather was fine the two men would walk together on the Terrace—a wide gravel path inside the asylum's south wall, shaded by tall old firs and araucaria, the monkey-puzzle tree. The lawns were green, the shrubbery filled with daffodils and tulips, and once in a while other patients would emerge from the blocks to play football, or walk, or sit staring into space from one of the wooden benches. Attendants would lurk in the shadows, making sure there were no outbreaks of trouble.

Murray and Minor, hands behind their backs, would walk in step, slowly back and forth along the three hundred yards of the Terrace, always in the shadows of either the gaunt red buildings or of the seventeen-foot wall. They always seemed animated, deep in conversation; papers were produced, sometimes books. They did not speak to others, and gave the impression of inhabiting a world of their own.

Sometimes Doctor Nicholson would invite the pair in for afternoon tea; and on one or two occasions Ada Murray came to Broadmoor too, and remained with Nicholson and his family in the superintendent's comfortably furnished house while the men pored over the books in the cell or on the gravel walkway. There was always sadness when the time came for the editor to leave: The keys would turn, the gates would clang shut, and Minor would be left alone again, trapped in a world of his own making, redeemed only when, after a day or so of quiet mourning, he could take down another volume from his shelves, select a needed word and its most elegant context, pick up his pen, and dip it in the ink to write once more: "To Dr. Murray, Oxford."

* * *

The Oxford Post Office knew the address well: It was all that was needed to communicate by letter with the greatest lexicographer in the land, and make sure the information got through to him at the Scriptorium.

Few enough letters between the two men survive. There is a lengthy letter from 1888, in which Minor writes about the quotations containing the word *chaloner*—an obsolete name for a man who manufactured shalloon, which was a woolen lining material for coats. He is interested, according to a later note, in the word *gondola*, and finds a quotation from Spenser, in 1590.

Murray talked about his new friend often, and liked to include him—and indeed, with some discreet reference to his condition—in the speeches he was often obliged to make. In 1897, for instance, his notes survive for a speech he was to give at a dictionary evening at the Philological Society: "About 15 or 16,000 add'l slips rec'd during the past year. Half of those supplied by Dr. W. C. Minor whose name and pathetic story, I have often before alluded to. Dr. M. has in reading 50 or 60 books, mostly scarce, of the 16th-17th C. His practice is to keep just ahead of the actual preparation of the Dictionary."

Two years later Murray felt able to be more fulsome still:

> The supreme position . . . is certainly held by Dr. W. C. Minor of Broadmoor, who during the past two years has sent in no less than 12,000 quots [*sic*]. These have nearly all been for the words which Mr.

Bradley and I were actually occupied, for Dr. Minor likes to know each month just what words we are likely to be working on during the month and to devote his whole strength to supplying quotations for those words, and thus to feel that he is in touch with the making of the Dictionary.

So enormous have been Dr. Minor's contributions during the past 17 or 18 years, that we could easily illustrate the last 4 centuries from his quotations alone. (Emphasis added.)

But the devotion of his whole strength was beginning to prove taxing, both to his body and his mind. His kindly friend Doctor Nicholson retired in 1895—still in pain from being attacked by a patient six years earlier, who hit him on the head with a brick concealed in a sock. He was replaced by Doctor Brayn, a man selected (for more than his name alone, one trusts) by a Home Office that felt a stricter regime needed to be employed at the asylum.

Brayn was indeed a martinet, a jailer of the old school who would have done well at a prison farm in Tasmania or Norfolk Island. But he did as the government required: There were no escapes during his term of office (there had been several before, causing widespread alarm), and in the first year two hundred thousand hours of solitary confinement were logged by the more fractious inmates. He was widely feared and loathed by the patients—as well as by Doctor Murray, who thought he was treating Minor heartlessly.

And Minor continues to whinge. He complains of a hole

in the heel of his sock, doubtless caused by some stranger's shoe into which, at night, he had been obliged to place his foot (November 1896). Minor is suspicious that his wines and spirits are being tampered with (December 1896).

One curious snippet of information came from the United States later that same year, when it was noted rather laconically that two of Minor's family had recently killed themselves—the letter going on to warn the staff at Broadmoor that great care should be taken lest whatever madness gripped their patient turned out to have a hereditary nature. But even if the staff thought Minor a possible suicide risk, no restrictions were placed on him as a result of the American information.

Some years before he had asked for a pocket knife, with which he might trim the uncut pages of some of the first editions of the books he had ordered: There is no indication that he was asked to hand it back, even with the harsh Doctor Brayn incharge. No other patient was allowed to keep a knife, but with his twin cells, his bottles, and his books, and with his part-time servant, William Minor seemed still to belong to a different category from most others in Broadmoor at the time.

In the year following the disclosure about his relatives, the files speak of Minor's having started to take walks out on the Terrace in all weathers, angrily denouncing those who tried to persuade him to come back in during one especially violent snowstorm, insisting in his imperious way that it was his business alone if he wished to catch cold. He had more freedom of choice and movement than most.

Not that this much improved his temper. A number of old army friends from America happened to come over to London in 1899, and all asked to come to Broadmoor. But the old officer refused to see any of them, saying he did not remember them, and besides, he did not want to be disturbed. He formally applied to be given some "freedom of the vicinage," to be let out on parole—the word he used being rather rare, and meaning essentially the same as "the vicinity."

The elegance of his language convinced no one, however, and his application was firmly denied. "He is still of unsound mind and I am unable to recommend that his request be granted," the superintendent wrote to the Home Secretary. (Or typed, it should be said: This is the first document in Minor's file that was produced on a typewriter—an indication that while the patient remained in a miserable stasis, the outside world around him was changing all too rapidly.) The Home Secretary duly then turned down the prayer; on the form is added a bleak initialed notation from the heartless Doctor Brayn: "Patient informed, 12.12.99. RB"

His diet ticket shows him to be eating fitfully—lots of porridge, sago pudding, custard every Tuesday, but bacon and other meat only occasionally. He appears to have become increasingly unhappy, troubled, listless. "He seems unsettled," is a constant theme of the attendants' notes. A visit from Murray in the summer of 1901 cheered him up, but soon afterward the staff at the dictionary were begin-

ning to notice a depressing change in their keenest surviv-
ing volunteer.

"I notice that he has sent no Q quotations," wrote Murray
to a friend.

> But he has been very slack altogether for many
> months, and I have scarcely heard anything from
> him. He always is less helpful in summer, because he
> spends so much more time in the open air, in the gar-
> den and grounds. But this year it is worse than usual,
> and I have been feeling for a good while that I shall
> have to take a day to go and see him again, and try to
> refresh his interest.
>
> In his lonely & sad position he requires a great
> deal of nursing, encouraging and coaxing, and I have
> had to go from time to time to see him.

A month later and things were no better. Murray wrote
about him again—by now there are stories of him "putting
his back up" and "refusing" to do the work that was wanted.
He wrote something about the origin of the word *hump*, as on
a camel—but aside from that, and coincident with the death
of Queen Victoria, he lapsed into a sullen silence.

Another old army friend writing from Northwich, in
Cheshire, in March 1902 asks Superintendent Brayn if he
might be allowed to visit Minor, telling him in some distress
that Minor himself had written saying that he ought not to,
since "things were much changed, and that I might find it un-

pleasant." Please give me your advice, the writer adds: "I do not wish to expose my wife to anything unpleasant."

Brayn agreed: "I do not think it would be advisable for you to visit . . . there are no indications of any immediate danger, but his years are beginning to tell on him . . . his life is precarious."

It was at about this time that there came the first indication that it might be better if Doctor Minor now be allowed to return to the United States, to spend his declining years—as he did seem to be in decline—close to his family.

Minor had been in Broadmoor now for thirty years—he was by far the longest-staying patient. He was sustained only by his books. Sadness had utterly enveloped him. He missed the ever-sympathetic Doctor Nicholson; he was perplexed by the more brutish regime of Doctor Brayn. His sole intellectual colleague among the Block 2 patients, the strange artist Richard Dadd, who had been sent to an asylum for stabbing dead his own father, had long since died. His own stepmother, Judith, whom he had seen briefly in 1885 on her way back from India, had died in New Haven in 1900. Age was fast winnowing out all those who were close to the mad old man.

Even old Fitzedward Hall had died, in 1901—an event that prompted Minor to fire off a letter of deep and abiding sadness to Murray. Along with his condolences went a request that the editor might perhaps enclose some more slips for the letters *K* and *O*—the news of the passing of his fellow countryman seems to have revived Minor's interest in work a little. But only a little. He was now quite alone, in worsening health, harmless to all but himself. He was sixty-six years old, and showing it. The facts of his circumstances were beginning to weigh heavily on him.

Dr. Francis Brown, the distinguished physician in Boston to whom Murray had written the full account of Minor and their first meeting, thought he might intervene. After hearing from Murray he had written to the Department of the Army in Washington and then to the American Embassy in London, and now in March to Doctor Brayn, suggesting that— without Minor's knowledge—a petition be sent to the Home Office asking for his release into his family's custody and his return to the United States. "His family would rejoice to have him spend his last days in his own land and nearer to them."

But the pitiless Brayn did not make the recommendation to the Home Secretary; and neither the embassy nor the U.S. Army chose to become involved. The old man was to stay put, encouraged only by the occasional correspondence from Oxford, but increasingly dispirited, angry, and sad.

A crisis was clearly about to erupt—and erupt it did. The event that in Hayden Church's orotund phrase "was the most striking feature in the American's history" struck without any warning that was heeded, on a cold morning at the beginning of December 1902.

10

The Unkindest Cut

Masturbate (mæ·stɒɹbeⁱt), *v.* [f. L. *masturbāt-*, ppl. stem of *masturbārī*, of obscure origin: according to Brugmann for **masturbārī* f. **mazdo-* (cf. Gr. μέξεα pl.) virile member + *turba* disturbance. An old conjecture regarded the word as f. *manu-s* hand + *stuprāre* to defile; hence the etymologizing forms MANUSTUPRATION, MASTUPRATE, -ATION, used by some Eng. writers.] *intr.* and *refl.* To practise self-abuse.

"At 10.55 am Dr. Minor came to the bottom gate, which was locked, and he called out: 'You had better send for the Medical Officer at once! I have injured myself!'"

The words are the first lines of a brief penciled note that lurks anonymously among the scores of other papers that measure out the trivial details of the life of Broadmoor's patient number 742. Reports of the more mundane features

of William Minor's now almost solitary life—his diet, his
steadily diminishing number of visitors, his growing frailty,
his curmudgeonly lapses, his insane ruminations—are usually made in ink, the writing steady and confident. But this
single page, which is dated December 3, 1902, is very different. The fact that it was written in thick pencil sets it apart—
but so does the handwriting, which makes it look as though it
was scrawled urgently, in a hurry, by a man who was breathless, panicky, in a state of shock.

Its author was the Block 2 principal attendant, a Mr.
Coleman. He had good reason to be appalled:

> I sent Attendant Harfield for the Medical Officer
> and went to see if I could assist Dr. Minor. Then he
> told me—he had cut his penis off. He said he had tied
> it with string, which had stopped the bleeding. I saw
> what he had done.
>
> Dr. Baker and Dr. Noott then saw him and he
> was removed to the B-3 Infirmary at 11.30am.
>
> He had taken his walk before breakfast as usual.
> Also he took his breakfast. I was talking to him at
> 9.50 in Ward 3, when he appeared to be just as usual.

But he was not in fact "just as usual"—whatever such a
phrase might mean in the context of his well-developed paranoia. Unless his act of self-mutilation was an extraordinary
reaction to some equally extraordinary event—which could
be the case, though there is no proof of it—it looks very much
as though William Minor had been planning it for several

days, if not for months. Cutting off his penis was, by his lights, a necessary and redemptive act: It had probably come about as the consequence of a profound religious awakening, which his doctors believed had begun two years before—or at the end of the century, thirty years after he had been committed.

Minor was the son of missionaries, and he had been brought up, at least notionally, as a staunch Congregationalist Christian. But while at Yale he had largely forsaken his religion, and by the time he was established in the Union army—whether he had become disillusioned by his experiences on the battlefield or simply uninterested in organized religion—he apparently abandoned his beliefs totally and was content to have himself described, without shame, as an atheist.

He was for a while a devoted reader of T. H. Huxley—the great Victorian biologist and philosopher who coined the term *agnostic*. His own feelings were more negative still: Since the laws of nature could quite satisfactorily explain all natural phenomena, he would write, he could not find any logical need for the existence of a God.

However, over the years in the asylum these feelings of hostility began slowly to ameliorate. By 1898 or so, his absolute certainty about the nonexistence of a God started to waver—perhaps in part because of the strong Christian beliefs of his frequent visitor James Murray, who was the object of Minor's intense and most lasting admiration. Murray may well have discussed the possible solace that Minor might gain from the recognition and acceptance of a superior divinity:

Unintentionally he may have triggered what turned out to be
Minor's steadily intensifying religious fervor.

By the turn of the century Minor had changed: He was
telling visitors, and formally informing the Broadmoor superintendent, that he now regarded himself as a deist—as
someone who accepts the existence of a God but does not sub-
scribe to any particular religion. It was an important step—
and yet, in its own way, it was a tragic one.

For in tandem with his new beliefs, Minor began to judge
himself by the harsh standards of what he believed to be an
all-purpose, all-seeing, and eternally vindictive deity. He
suddenly stopped thinking of his insanity as a treatable sadness and instead took to thinking of it—or of some of its aspects—as an intolerable affliction, a state of sin that needed
constant purging and punishment. He began to regard himself not as a sorry creature, but as someone inexpressibly vile,
endowed with dreadful habits and leanings. He was a com-
pulsive and obsessive masturbator. God would be certain to
punish him dreadfully should he fail to halt his wholesale
dependence on self-abuse.

His prodigious sexual appetites in particular started to become particularly abhorrent to him: He began to be haunted
by the memory—or the fantastic supposed memory—of his
past sexual conquests. He began to loathe the way his body responded, and with the way that God had so inappropriately
and unjustly equipped him. As his medical file reported:

> He believed there had been a complete saturation
> of his entire being with the lasciviousness of over 20

years, during which time he had relations with thousands of nude women, night after night. The nightly dissipations had had no perceptible influence on his physical strength, but his organ had increased in size as the result of such constant use, his constant priapism had allowed it to develop enormously. He remembers a Frenchwoman remarking "bien fait!" on first seeing it; another woman had called him "an apostle of pleasure"; sexual adventure and fantasy gave him as much pleasure as anything else in the world.

But when he became Christianized he saw that he must sever himself from the lascivious life that he had been leading—and decided that the amputation of his penis would solve the problem.

The surgical removal of the penis is at the best of times a dangerous practice, rarely performed even by doctors: An attack by the renowned Brazilian fishlet known as *candiru*, which likes to swim up a man's urine stream and lodge in the urethra with a ring of retrorse spines preventing its removal, is one of the very rare circumstances in which doctor will perform the operation, known as a peotomy. It is a brave, foolhardy, and desperate man who will perform an autopeotomy, in which one removes one's own organ—the more so when the operation is done in an unsterile environment and with a pen knife.

Among his many perks, as we have seen, Doctor Minor had enjoyed—unlike all the other Broadmoor patients—the superintendent's permission to carry a pen knife. It had long ceased to be of much use: Few were the occasions when he had to cut the unfinished pages of first editions, which is why he had asked for the knife in the first place. Now it just sat in his pocket, as it might in that of an ordinary man on the outside world. Except that Minor was in no sense ordinary—and he now had, it turned out, an unusual and pressing need for the knife.

He was desperately certain that it was his penis that had led him to commit all the unsavory deeds that had so dominated his life. His continuing sexual desires, if not born in his penis, were at least carried out by it. In his delusional world he felt he had no alternative but to remove it. He was a doctor, of course, and so knew roughly what he was doing.

So on that Wednesday morning he sharpened his knife on a whetstone. He tied a thin cord tightly around the base of his member to act as a ligature and to pressure-cauterize the blood vessels, he waited for ten minutes or so until the vein and artery walls had become properly compressed—and then, in one swift movement that most would prefer not to imagine, he sliced off his organ about one inch from its base.

He threw the offending object into the fire. He relaxed the string and found that, as he had expected, there was almost no blood. He lay down for a while to ensure there was no hemorrhage and then walked almost casually to the lower gate on the ground floor of Block 2 and called for the attendant. His training taught him he would probably now go into shock, and he supposed that he needed to be put into the asylum infirmary—as indeed the astonished Broadmoor doctors ordered.

He remained there for the best part of a month—and within days was displaying his old cantankerous self, complaining at the noise the workmen were making, even though the day he chose to complain was a Sunday, when the workmen were all at home.

The penis steadily healed, leaving a small stump through which Minor could urinate, but that—to his presumed satisfaction—proved to be useless sexually. The problem had been solved: The Deity would be satisfied that no further sexual rompings could take place. The doctor remarked in his ward notes that he was amazed that anyone had had the nerve to perform such an extraordinary mutilation on himself.

There remains one further possible reason for his having carried out so bizarre an act—a reason that some might think rather stretches credulity. He may have amputated his penis out of guilt and self-loathing for having enjoyed either some kind of relationship with, or lascivious thoughts about, the widow of the man he had murdered.

Eliza Merrett, it will be remembered, had visited Minor at the asylum at regular intervals in the early 1880s. She used to bring books and occasional gifts; he and his stepmother had given her money as recompense for her loss; she had said, quite publicly, that she had forgiven him for the murder; she had accepted, and sympathetically, that he had committed the crime while not knowing right from wrong. Might it not have been possible that in a moment of mutual consolation something passed between these two people—who were almost the same age, and who in many senses were similarly reduced in circumstances? And might it not be that one day, eventually, the memory of the event plunged the sensitive and thoughtful Doctor Minor into a deep and guilt-ridden depression?

No suggestion exists that the meetings between Minor and Eliza Merrett were anything other than proper, formal, and chaste—and perhaps they always were so, and any residual guilt that Minor may have felt stemmed from the kind of fantasies to which his medical records show him to have been prey. But it has to be admitted that it remains a possibility—not a probability, to be sure—that it was guilt for a specific act, rather than some slow-burning religious fervor, that prompted this horrible tragedy.

It was exactly a year afterward that the question of removing Doctor Minor to the United States was raised once again. This time his brother Alfred, who was still running the china emporium back in New Haven, suggested it in a private letter to the superintendent, which Minor never saw. This time, and for the first time, the usually rebarbative Doctor Brayn offered some grounds for hope: "[I]f arrangements could be made for his proper care and treatment, and if the American government would agree to his removal, I think it is quite possible that the proposal might be favourably considered."

A year later still and James Murray visited, on his way back home from seeing his daughter at college in London. He told Brayn that Minor was "my friend," and said later he was distressed at how frail he seemed, at how the light and energy that had marked him in his dictionary-busy days of the previous decade seemed now to have deserted him. Murray was further convinced that the old gentleman must be allowed to go home to die. In England he had no one and no work, no reason for existence. His life was merely a slow-moving tragedy, an act of steady dying conducted before everyone's eyes.

William Minor repaid the pleasure of the visit in an unusually intimate way: He gave him a small amount of money. James Murray was going off to the Cape Colony—part of what is now South Africa—to attend a conference, and somehow Minor discovered that it was a journey that would stretch Murray's finances to the limit (though the normally parsimonious Oxford University Press Delegates gave him a hundred pounds). So Minor decided to pitch in as well, and sent out for a postal order for a few pounds, which he sent along with a curiously affectionate note, as one elder might write to another:

> Pray pardon the liberty I take, to enclose you a postal payable to your order—that I thought might add in a small way against unexpected demands upon your means.
>
> Even a *millionaire* may feel satisfaction to find he has a sovereign more than he thought for, though himself a republican, and we less gifted people have a right to a like satisfaction when the chance permits.
>
> Building a house and going on a journey are much the same, in costing more than one expects; and in any case I am sure you can make this useful.

Now I will say goodbye to you both, with best
wishes for your welfare, and in its uncontracted form
also,

God be with you,
W. C. Minor

And over the succeeding weeks and months, the insane
man became steadily the infirm man. He fell in his bath; he
hurt his leg; he tripped and twisted leathery sinews and weary
muscles; he suffered from the cold, and he caught a chill. All
the casual inconveniences of old age were being piled onto
his madness, each a Pelion upon Ossa, until William Minor
was no more than a thin and elderly wretch, feared by no one,
pitied by all.

Then there came a pathetic example of a smaller madness. Though no longer much of a lexicographer or a flutist,
Doctor Minor remained something of a painter, and filled
many hours working at the easel set up in his room. One day,
on a whim, he decided he would send one of his better works
to the Princess of Wales, the young woman—May of Teck,
Queen Mary to be—who was wife of the man who would
soon become King George V.

But Doctor Brayn said no. Bleakly and predictably enforc-
ing the rule that no inmate at Broadmoor may communicate
with any member of the royal family—a rule made because
so many deranged inmates supposed themselves to *be* members of the royal family—he told Minor that he could not
send it. The doctor, angry and querulous, then formally ap-
pealed, forcing Brayn to send the painting and a petition to

the Home Office, whose minister had the ultimate say. The office not unnaturally backed Brayn, and Brayn wrote again to Minor, denying his petition.

But this caused Minor to get his dander up, and he wrote furiously and barely legibly to the American ambassador, asking that he use his good diplomatic offices to transmit the package to Buckingham Palace. The package was never sent: Brayn insisted that he would not allow it. So Minor sent a further letter to the U.S. Army Chief of Staff in Washington, complaining that he, an officer in the U.S. Army himself, was being forcibly prevented from communicating with his embassy.

The whole saga became then the focus of a long summer month's work by a host of attachés and vice-consuls and heads of protocol and assistants to senior staff officers, all bickering and wondering whether this harmless old man's doubtless charming watercolor could ever find its way into the hands of the Princess of Wales.

But it never did. Permission was denied up and down the line—and the whole episode ended in a melancholy way. For when Doctor Minor sadly retreated to his cell block and asked plaintively for his painting back, he was informed with cold hauteur that it had in fact been lost. The letter asking for the painting back is in a spidery, shaky hand—the hand of an elderly, half sane, half senile man—and it was to no avail. The painting has never been recovered.

And there were further dispiriting developments. In early March 1910, Doctor Brayn—whom history will probably not judge kindly in the specific case of William Minor—

ordered that all the old man's privileges be taken away. Minor was given just a day's notice to quit the suite of two rooms that he had occupied for the previous thirty-seven years, to leave behind his volumes of books, to give up his access to his writing table, his sketchpads and his flutes, and move into the asylum infirmary. It was a cruel outrage committed by a vengeful man, quite likely jealous of the burgeoning reputation of his charge, and angry letters poured in from the few remaining friends who heard the news.

Even Ada Murray—now Lady Murray, since James had been knighted in 1908, recommended by a grateful Prime Minister Herbert Asquith—complained bitterly on her husband's behalf about the cruel and cavalier treatment that was apparently being meted out to the seventy-six-year-old Minor. Brayn replied limply: "I should not have curtailed any of his privileges had I not been convinced that to leave things as they were was running the risk of a serious accident."

But neither Sir James nor Lady Murray was mollified: It was imperative, they said, that their scholar-genius friend now be allowed to go home to America, out of the clutches of this monstrous Doctor Brayn, and away from a hospital that no longer seemed the benign home of harmless scholarship but more closely resembled the Bedlam it had once been constructed to replace.

Minor's brother Alfred sailed to London in late March with a view to resolving the situation once and for all. He had spoken to the U.S. Army in Washington; the generals there said it was possible, providing only that the British Home Office agreed, to have Doctor Minor transferred to the place in which he had been incarcerated very many years before—St. Elizabeth's Federal Hospital in the American capital. If Alfred agreed to keep his brother in safe custody for the transfer across the Atlantic, then it might well be possible to persuade the home secretary to issue the requisite permission.

Fate was to intervene in a merciful way. By great good fortune the home secretary of the day was Winston Churchill—a man who, though less well known then than he would soon become, had a naturally sympathetic inclination toward Americans, since his mother was one. He ordered his civil servants to send a summary of the case up to his office—a summary that still exists, and offers a concise and intriguing indication of how governments manage their business.

The various arguments for and against the parole of Doctor Minor are offered; the decision is deemed ultimately to rest only on whether, if Minor is still judged to be a danger to others, his brother Alfred can really be trusted to keep him away from firearms during any transfer. The bureaucrats working on the case then slowly but inexorably come to parallel understandings—that on the one hand Minor is not dangerous, and that on the other his brother could be well trusted, if need be. So the recommendation made to Churchill on the basis of this turgid process of exposition and analysis was that the man should indeed be released on parole and allowed to go off to his native land.

And so, on Wednesday, April 6, 1910, Winston S. Churchill duly signed, in blue ink, a Warrant of Conditional Discharge, subject only to the condition that Minor "shall on his discharge leave the United Kingdom and not return thereto."

The next day Sir James Murray wrote, asking if he might be allowed to say good-bye to his old friend and if he might bring Lady Murray as well. "There is not the least objection," said Doctor Brayn, smoothly, "and he is in much better health, and will be pleased to see you." One can almost hear the lifting of the old man's spirits with the thought that after thirty-eight long years, he was finally going home.

Since the occasion was a momentous one—both for Minor and for England, in more ways than could be immediately understood—Murray had invited an artist from Messrs. Russell & Co., Photographers to His Majesty the King, to take a formal farewell portrait of Doctor Minor, in the Broadmoor asylum garden. Doctor Brayn said he had no objection; the picture that resulted remains a most sympathetic portrait of a kindly, scholarly, and from his facial expression, not un-content figure, seemingly seated after tea under a peaceful English hedgerow, unconstrained, untroubled, careless of everything.

At dawn on Saturday, April 16, 1910, Principal Attendant Spanholtz—a lot of Broadmoor attendants were, like him, Boer former prisoners of war—was ordered to proceed on escort duty, "in plain clothes," to escort William Minor to London. Sir James and Lady Murray were there in the weak spring sun to say farewell: There were formal handshakes and, it is said, the glistening of tears.

But these were more dignified times than our own; and the two men who had meant so very much to each other for so long, and the creation of whose combined scholarship was now almost half complete—the six so-far-published volumes of the *OED* were packed securely in Minor's valise—said good-bye to each other in an air of stiff formality. Doctor Brayn offered his own curt valedictory, and the landau rattled its way down the lanes, soon becoming lost to view in an early spring mist. Two hours later it was at Bracknell Station, on the South East Main Line to London.

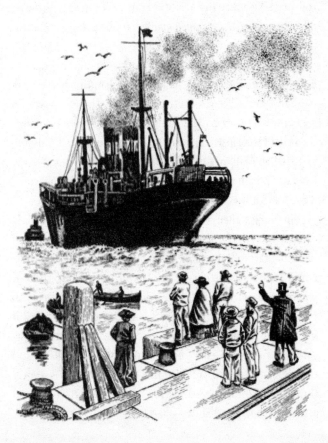

An hour later Spanholtz and Minor were at the mighty, vaulting cathedral of Waterloo Station—much larger than it had been when, no more than a few hundred yards away, the murder that began this story was committed on that Saturday night in 1872. The pair did not linger, for obvious reasons, but took a hansom cab to St. Pancras Station and there caught the boat train to Tilbury Docks. They walked to the quayside where the Atlantic Transport Line's twin-screw passenger liner S.S. *Minnetonka* lay, coaling and victualing, bound that afternoon for New York.

It was only at dockside that the Broadmoor attendant finally relinquished custody of his charge, handing him over to Alfred Minor, who was waiting beside the ship's gangway. A receipt was duly offered and signed, just before noon, as though the patient were just a large box or a haunch of meat. "This is to certify that William Chester Minor has this day been received from the Broadmoor Criminal Lunatic Asylum into my care," it read, and it was signed, "Alfred W. Minor, Conservator."

Spanholtz then waved his own cheery good-bye, and raced off to catch his return train. At two o'clock the vessel blasted a farewell on its steam horn and, with tugs yelping, edged out into the estuary of the Thames. By midafternoon it was off the landmark lighthouse on the Kentish coast's North Foreland and had turned hard to starboard; by nightfall it was in the Channel; by dawn on the next fresh morning, south of the Scilly Isles, and by lunchtime all England and the nightmare that it enfolded had finally receded, lost, over the damp taffrail. The sea was gray and huge and empty, and ahead lay the United States—and home.

Two weeks later Doctor Brayn received a note from New Haven.

> I am glad to say that my brother safely made the trip, and is now pleasantly fixed in the St. Elizabeth's Asylum in Washington DC. He enjoyed the voyage very much and had no trouble from sea-sickness. I thought he walked about too much for the latter part of the voyage. He did not trouble me at night— though I felt much relief on arriving at the dock in New York. . . . I hope I have the pleasure of meeting you at some future date. My regards to yourself and your family, and best wishes to all the Broadmoor staff and attendants.

11

Then Only the Monuments

Diagnosis (dəĭĕgn*ō*ᵘ·sis). Pl. **-oses**. [a. L. diagn*ō*sis, Gr. διάγνωσις, n. of action f. διαγιγνώσκειν to distinguish, discern, f. δια- through, thoroughly, asunder + γιγνώσκειν to learn to know, perceive. In F. *diagnose* in Molière: cf. prec.]

1. *Med.* Determination of the nature of a diseased condition; identification of a disease by careful investigation of its symptoms and history; also, the opinion (formally stated) resulting from such investigation.

Old Frederick Furnivall was the first of the great dictionary men to go. He died within just a few weeks of the *Minnetonka's* sailing from London.

Furnivall had known he was dying since the beginning of that fateful year, 1910. He remained amusing and energetic to the end, sculling his little boat at Hammersmith, flirting with his waitresses at the ABC, sending his daily packages

of words and newspaper clippings to the editor of a project
with which he had been intimately associated for all of half
of a century.

He started one of his final letters to Murray with a typically eccentric disdain for the illness that he knew would
shortly fell him. His first expressed interest was in a word—
tallow-catch—that Murray had found in Shakespeare, had
recently defined, and had sent down to Hammersmith for
approval: Furnivall offered his congratulations for a definition that read in part "a very fat man . . . a tub of tallow," a
word that has similarities today with the reference to a man
as "a tub of lard." Only after this did he speak elliptically of
the grim prognosis his doctor had offered—he had intestinal
cancer—remarking, "Yes, our Dict. Men go gradually, & I am
to disappear in six months. . . . It's a great disappointment, as
I wanted to see the Dict. finished before I die. But it is not to
be. However the completion of the word is certain. So that's
all right."

He died as predicted, in July; but he did not abandon
work until after inspecting, as Murray had suggested that he
might, one majestically long entry that was due for inclusion
in volume 11. "Would it give you any satisfaction," Murray
had asked him, "to see the gigantic TAKE in final? Before it
is too late?"

Murray himself, given his steadily advancing years, suspected that with Furnivall's passing, his own end could not
be too far off. And with offering *take* to Furnivall it was evident he had only just begun the monumental work on the
entirety of the letter *T*. That single letter was to take him five

long years—from 1908 until 1913—to complete. When he finished he was so relieved as to voice an incautiously optimistic forecast: "I have got to the stage where I can estimate the end. In all human probability *the Oxford English Dictionary* will be finished on my eightieth birthday, four years from now."

But it was not to be. Neither was the *OED* to be completed in four years, nor was Sir James ever to become an octogenarian. The grand conjunction for which he hoped—his own golden wedding anniversary, his dictionary's completion—never happened. Oxford's Regius Professor of Medicine once joked that the university seemed to be paying him a salary "just to keep that old man alive" so he can complete his work. They did not, it seems, pay enough.

His prostate gave up on him in the spring of 1915, and the burning X rays with which such problems were then treated hurt him severely. He kept up his pace of work, completing *trink* to *turndown* in mid-summer, and including many difficult words that, as a fellow editor said, "were handled with characteristic sagacity and resource." He was photographed for the last time in the Scriptorium on July 10—his staff and daughters around and behind him, and in the background shelves of bound books replacing the pigeonholes with their thousands of slips of paper, which had been the familiar backdrop in the dictionary's earlier days. His academic cap still atop his head, Sir James looks thin and weary; his expression is one of calm resignation, those of the people beside him knowing and tragic.

He died on July 26, 1915, of pleurisy, and was buried as

he wished to be, beside a great Oxford friend who had been professor of Chinese.

William Minor, now into his fifth year at the Government Hospital for the Insane in Washington, D.C.—which was known until 1916 only informally by its later permanent name, St. Elizabeth's—would have heard in due course of the death of the man who had brought him so much solace and intellectual comfort. But on the actual day of Murray's passing, he merely had yet another of the bad days that he was increasingly now enduring. Some might say that it was a day on which Minor in Washington was unknowingly in sympathy with the sad events that were unfolding in Oxford, more than three thousand miles across the Atlantic Ocean.

"Struck one of his fellow-patients," read the notes of Minor's Cherry Ward for that same Monday evening, July 26. "He had happened to stop and look into his room. Shows temper and will try to strike hard, but has little strength to hurt anyone." (He had started hitting people the month before. He went walking one June afternoon, along with his attendant, and the pair met a policeman. When the officer began to ask questions, Minor started pounding the attendant on the chest—though he later said he was sorry, explaining that he was becoming "a little excitable.")

He had probably been capable of inflicting little hurt from the moment he was first entered in the hospital log. He may have been mad, but he was painfully slender; his spine was bowed; he shuffled as he walked; he had lost his teeth and had alopecia. Photographs were taken, full-front and in

profile, as if he were a common criminal: His beard is long
and white, his bald head high and domed, his eyes wild. His
madness was defined as simple paranoia, the doctors said; he
admitted that he still thought constantly about little girls,
and that he had dreams about the appalling acts they had
made him perform during his forced nightly excursions.

But he was not regarded as dangerous: His doctors agreed
that he should be granted the privilege of walking into the
surrounding countryside, if accompanied by an attendant.
The stump of his penis attested dramatically to the fact that
he should not be allowed access either to a knife or to scis-
sors. But otherwise, he was deemed harmless—he was just
a seventy-seven-year-old man, thin, toothless, wrinkled,
slightly deaf, yet "very active, considering his age."

His delusions steadily worsened during the St. Elizabeth's
years. He complained that his eyes were regularly pecked out
by birds, that people forced food into his mouth through a
metal funnel and then hammered on his fingernails, that
scores, of pygmies hid beneath the floorboards of his room
and acted as agents for the underworld. He was occasionally
irritable but more usually quiet and courteous, and he read
and wrote a great deal in his room. He had a somewhat arrogant air, said one doctor: He did not much care for the company of his fellow patients, and he would absolutely not let
any one of them come into his private room.

It was at St. Elizabeth's that his hitherto puzzling illness
was given what might be regarded as its first modern, currently recognizable description. On November 8, 1918, his
attending psychiatrist, a Doctor Davidian, formally declared

that William Minor, federal patient number 18487, was suffering from what was to be called "dementia praecox, of the paranoid form." No longer was the vague word *monomania* to be used, nor would simple *paranoia* do. Minor and his case history had finally been cast off from the dubious moorings of the Victorians' puzzled but determinedly "moral treatment" of the mad—the phrase had been coined by the Frenchman Philippe Pinel of the Salpêtrière hospital in Paris—and were at last to be welcomed into the world of modern psychiatry.

The new phrase, *dementia praecox*, was quite precise. By the time Davidian employed it as a diagnosis it had been current for twenty years. It literally meant early-flowering failure of the mental powers, and was used to distinguish a condition in which a person begins to lose touch with reality, as Minor had done, early on his life—in his teens, his twenties, or his thirties. In this sense the illness was markedly different from *senile dementia*, a term once used to describe the decrepitude that specifically accompanies old age, and of which Alzheimer's disease is one kind.

The nomenclature was published in Heidelberg in 1899 by the German psychiatrist Emil Kraepelin, who at the time was the supreme classifier of known mental ills. His naming of the condition was designed less to distinguish it from being an old person's ailment as to mark it as very different from manic-depressive psychosis, an illness that had enough similarities to confuse the earliest of the alienists.

Kraepelin's view, revolutionary at the time, was that while manic-depressive psychoses had identifiable physical causes (such as a low level of the alkaline metal lithium in the blood and brain), and were thus treatable (as with the use of lithium pills, for example, to make up a depressive's lack of it), dementia praecox was a so-called endogenous ailment, quite lacking in any identifiable external cause. In that respect it was to be regarded as similar to such enigmatic systemic physical disorders as essential hypertension, in which a patient develops high blood pressure—and its many untidy and inconvenient side effects—for no obvious reason.

Kraepelin went on to define three distinct subtypes of dementia praecox. There was catatonic, in which the motor functions of the body are either excessive or nonexistent; hebephrenic, in which grotesquely inappropriate behavior begins during puberty, hence the word's origin from the Greek ήβη "youth"; and paranoiac, in which the victim suffers from delusions, often of persecution. It was from this kind of dementia, according to Kraepelin's classification of the time, that Doctor Minor was suffering.

The traditional treatment offered to him and his kind was still simple, basic, and by today's standards, dismayingly unenlightened. Those suffering from paranoid dementia were deemed pathologically incurable, were removed from society by court order, and were placed—kindly, tenderly, for the most part, thanks to Pinel's powerful influence—in cells behind high walls, so as to cause no inconvenience to those living in the normal, outside world. Some were incarcerated for only a very few years; some for ten or twenty. In the case of Minor his involuntary exile from society was to last for most of his life. He existed for most of his first thirty-eight years on the outside, until he killed George Merrett. Then, for forty-seven of the forty-eight years that were left to him, he was locked away in state asylums, essentially untreated because he was, in the view of the doctors of the day, essentially untreatable.

Since the time of Minor and Davidian, the illness has become much more liberally regarded. Its name, for a start, has changed: What was initially the far less daunting word *schizophrenia*—it came from the Greek for "split mind"—made its first appearance in 1912. (It may change again: To rid the ailment of its patina of unpleasant associations, there are now moves—perhaps not entirely prudent—to have it called Kraepelin's syndrome.)

Early treatments for the disease, which were just being introduced at the time of Minor's final decline, involved the use of massive sedatives like chloral hydrate, sodium amytal, and paraldehyde. Today entire shelves of costly antipsychotic drugs are available at least to treat and manage schizophrenia's more discomfiting symptoms. But so far, and despite the spending of fortunes, there have been precious few advances in staying the mysterious triggers that seemingly set off the illness and its demonic mischiefs.

And there continues to be much debate about what these triggers might be. Can it ever be said that a major psychological illness like schizophrenia, with its severe disruption of the brain's chemistry, appearance, and function, truly has a *cause*? In the case of William Minor, could the terrible scenes at the Battle of the Wilderness actually have triggered his florid behavior?

Might his branding of an Irishman have precipitated, led

directly, or contributed even indirectly, to the crime he committed eight years later, which led to the exile he was to suffer
for the remainder of his life? Was there ever an identifiable
happening, had he ever been exposed to the mental equivalent of an invading germ? Or is schizophrenia truly causeless,
a part of the very being of some unfortunate individuals?
Moreover, what *is* the illness—is it simply the development
of a personality that is several steps beyond mere eccentricity,
and that steps into areas society does not find itself able to
tolerate or approve?

No one is quite certain. In 1984 a paper was presented
describing a man who firmly believed himself to have two
heads. He found one of them irritating beyond endurance,
and shot at it with a revolver, injuring himself terribly in the
process. He was diagnosed as schizophrenic, and the psychiatric community agreed, since it was manifestly certain that
the man only had one head, and suffered from and was dominated by an absurd delusion. But then again, the notorious
"Mad Lucas" of Victorian Hertfordshire, who lived with his
wife's dead body for three months and then by himself, in
wild biblical solitude and squalor for the next quarter century, and was visited by coachloads of day-trippers up from
London—he was diagnosed as schizophrenic too. Should
he have been? Was he not merely a borderline eccentric, be-
having in a fashion beyond the accepted norms? Was he as
mad as the deluded owner of the phantom head? Was he as
dangerous, and as deserving of confinement? And how does
a case like William Minor's sit within the spectrum of this
madness? Was he less mad than the first man, and more so

than the second? How does one quantify? How does one treat? How does one judge?

Psychiatrists today remain cautious about all of these questions, and puzzled and argumentative about whether the illness can be triggered—does have a definable cause. Most academic psychiatrists hedge their bets, avoiding dogma, preferring simply to say that they believe in the cumulative effect of a number of factors.

A patient may have a simple genetic predisposition to the illness. Or characteristics of the person's basic temperament may similarly increase the likelihood that he or she will "react badly" or floridly to an external stress—to the sights of a battlefield, to the shock of a torture, for example. And then again, maybe certain sights and the shocks are too great, or too sudden, for anyone to endure them and remain wholly sane.

There is the recently recognized condition known as posttraumatic stress disorder, which seems to affect inordinately large numbers of people who have been exposed to truly appalling situations. The only difference between their cases today, after the Gulf War, where it was first identified en masse, or after the trauma of a kidnap or a traffic accident, is that most sufferers are relieved of their symptoms after a period of time. But William Chester Minor never was. His agony endured for his entire life. However convenient it may be to say that posttraumatic stress ruined his life—and that of his victim—the continuing symptoms suggest otherwise. There was something wildly wrong with his brain, and what happened in Virginia probably prompted its more ruinous manifestations to emerge.

Perhaps it was an unusual genetic makeup that predisposed him to fall ill—two of his relations had killed themselves, after all, though we are not certain of the circumstances. Maybe his gentle temperament—he was a painter, a flutist, a collector of old books—made him unusually vulnerable to what he saw and felt on those blood-soaked fields in the South. Maybe his subsequent imprisonment in Broadmoor then left him unimproved, when a more compassionate and enlightened regime might have mitigated his darker feelings, might have helped him recover. One in a hundred people today suffer from schizophrenia: Nearly all of them, if treated with compassion and good chemistry, can have some kind of dignified life, of a kind that was denied, for much of his time, to Doctor Minor.

Except, of course, that Minor had his dictionary work. And there is a cruel irony in this—that if he *had* been so treated, he might never have felt impelled to work on it as he did. By offering him mood-altering sedatives, as they would have done in Edwardian times, or treating him as today with such antipsychotic drugs as quetiapine or risperidone, many of his symptoms of madness might have gone away—but he might well have felt disinclined or unable to perform his work for Doctor Murray.

In a sense doing all those dictionary slips *was* his medication; in a way they became his therapy. The routine of his quiet and cellbound intellectual stimulus, month upon month, year upon year, appears to have provided him with at least a measure of release from his paranoia. His sad situation only worsened when that stimulus was gone: when the great book ceased to function as his lodestone, when the one fixed point on which his remarkable but tortured brain was able to concentrate became detached, so then he began to spiral downward, and his life began to ebb.

One must feel a sense of strange gratitude, then, that his treatment was never good enough to divert him from his work. The agonies that he must have suffered in those terrible asylum nights have granted us all a benefit, for all time. He was mad, and for that, we have reason to be glad. A truly savage irony, on which it is discomfiting to dwell.

In November 1915, four months after Sir James had died, Doctor Minor wrote to Lady Murray in Oxford, offering her all the books that had been sent from Broadmoor to the Scriptorium, and that had been in Sir James's possession when he died. He hoped they might eventually go off to the Bodleian Library. "I am glad . . . to know that you are well, as I must presume from your letter and occupations. You must be taking or giving a great deal of labour for Dict'y materials still . . ." He uses the English spellings of words: Clearly his years in Broadmoor had left their mark in more ways than the merely custodial.

And his books do indeed rest in the great library to this day: They are registered as having been donated "By Dr. Minor through Lady Murray."

But by now he was failing steadily. An old colleague from Civil War days wrote from West Chester, Pa., to ask how his friend was—and the hospital superintendent replies that, considering his years, Captain Minor is in good health, and is in a "bright and cheerful ward, where he seems contented with his surroundings."

But the ward notes tell a different story, presenting as they do a litany of all the symptoms of the steady onset of senility and dementia. With increasing frequency the attendants write of Minor stumbling, injuring himself, getting lost, losing his temper, wandering, growing dizzy, tiring easily—and worst of all, beginning to forget, and knowing that he was forgetting. His mind, though tortured, had always been peculiarly acute: Now, by 1918 and the end of World War I, he seemed to know that his faculties were dimming, that his mind was at last becoming as weakened as his body, and that the sands were running out. For days at a time he would stay in bed, saying he needed "a good rest": He would barricade the door with chairs, still certain he was being persecuted. It was more than forty-five years since the murder, fully half a century since the first signs of madness had been noticed, back at the Florida army fort. And yet still the symptoms remained the same—persistent, uncured, incurable.

Still came the occasional querulous note, such as this, written in the summer of 1917:

> Dr. White—Dear Sir, There was a time when the meat—beef and ham—was very tough and dry. This has in a degree altered for the better since your note even, and I would not complain of that; and rice seemed to be the only vegetable with it.

This is not much to complain of; and yet these trifles are much to us in this life.

Thanking you for what you would wish to do.

I am very truly yours

W. C. Minor

A year later—though his failing memory and eyesight cause him to date the letter 1819 rather than 1918—he shows another strange spurt of benevolence, similar to his contributing to James Murray's adventure to the Cape. In this latest case he sent twenty-five dollars to the Belgian Relief Fund, and a further twenty-five to Yale University, his alma mater, as a donation to its military service fund. The president of Yale wrote back from Woodbridge Hall: "I have known much of Dr. Minor's history," he replied to the superintendent, "and am therefore doubly touched to receive this gift."

In 1919 his nephew Edward Minor applied to the army to have him released from St. Elizabeth's and brought to a hospital for the elderly insane in Hartford, Conn., known as The Retreat. The army agreed—"I think if the Retreat fully understands the case we should let him go," said a Doctor Duval at an October conference to discuss the matter. "He is getting so old now he will probably not do much harm." The hospital board agreed too, and in November, in a snowstorm, the frail old gentleman left Washington, and the strange world of insane asylums—a world that he had inhabited since 1872—for good and for ever.

* * *

He liked his new home, a mansion set in acres of woods and gardens on the banks of the Connecticut River. His nephew wrote in the early winter of 1920 of how the change seemed to have done him some good; and yet at the same time how incapable he was of looking after himself. Furthermore, he was fast going blind and for some months had been unable to read. With this one overarching source of joy now denied to him, there must have seemed to him little left to live for. No one was surprised when, after a walk on a blustery early spring day in that same year, he caught a cold that turned into bronchopneumonia, and died peacefully in his sleep. It was Friday, March 26, 1920. He had lived for eighty-five years and nine months. He might have been mad, but like Doctor Johnson's dictionary elephant, he had been "extremely long lifed."

There were no obituaries: just two lines in the Deaths columns of the *New Haven Register*. He was taken down to his old hometown and buried in the Evergreen Cemetery on the afternoon of the following Monday, in the family plot that had been established by his missionary father, Eastman Strong Minor. The gravestone is small and undistinguished, made of reddish sandstone, and bears only his name, William Chester Minor. An angel stands on a plinth nearby, gazing skyward, with the engraved motto, My Faith Looks Up to Thee.

Around the Evergreen Cemetery a high chain-link fence keeps out an angry part of New Haven, well away from the stern elegance of Yale. The simple existence of the fence un-

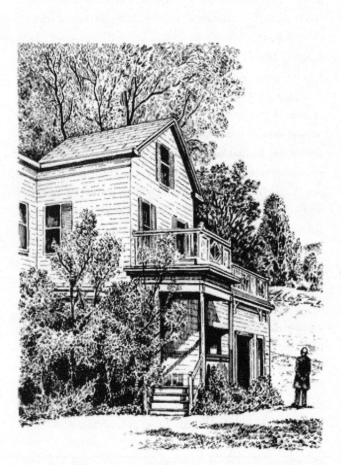

derlines a sad and ironic reality: Dr. William Minor, who was among the greatest of contributors to the finest dictionary in all the English language, died forgotten in obscurity, and is buried beside a slum.

The *Oxford English Dictionary* itself took another eight years to finish, the announcement of its completion made on New Year's Eve, 1927. The *New York Times* put the fact on the front page the next morning, a Sunday—that with the inclusion of the Old Kentish word *zyxt*—the second indicative present tense, in local argot, of the verb *to see*—the work was done, the alphabet was exhausted, and the full text was now wholly in the printers' hands. The making of the great book, declared the newspaper roundly and generously, was "one of the great romances of English literature."

The Americans did indeed love the story of its making. H. L. Mencken—no mean lexicographer himself—wrote that he fully expected Oxford to celebrate the culmination of the seventy-year project with "military exercises, boxing matches between the dons, orations in Latin, Greek, English and the Oxford dialect, yelling matches between the different Colleges and a series of medieval drinking bouts." Considering that the final editor of the book was dividing his time between professorships at both Oxford and Chicago, there was more than good reason for Americans to take a keen interest in a creation that was now, at least partly, of their own making.

The lonely drudgery of lexicography, the terrible undertow of words against which men like Murray and Minor had so ably struggled and stood, now had at last its great reward. Twelve mighty volumes; 414,825 words defined; 1,827,306 illustrative quotations used, to which William Minor alone had contributed scores of thousands.

The total length of type—all hand-set, for the books were done by letterpress, still discernible in the delicately impressed feel of the inked-on paper—is 178 miles, the distance between London and the outskirts of Manchester. Discounting every punctuation mark and every space—which any printer knows occupy just as much time to set as does a single letter—there are no fewer than 227,779,589 letters and numbers.

Other dictionaries in other languages took longer to make; but none was greater, grander, or had more authority than this. The greatest effort since the invention of printing. The longest sensational serial ever written.

One word—and only one word—was ever actually lost: *bondmaid*, which appears in Johnson's dictionary, was actually mislaid by Murray and was found, a stray without a home, long after the fascicle *Battentlie-Bozzom* had been published. It, and tens of thousands of words that had evolved or appeared during the forty-four years spent assembling the fascicles and their parent volumes, appeared in a supplement, which came out in 1933. Four further supplements appeared between 1972 and 1986. In 1989, using the new abilities of the computer, Oxford University Press issued its fully integrated second edition, incorporating all the changes and additions of the supplements in twenty rather more slender volumes. To help boost sales in the late seventies a two-volume set in a much-reduced typeface was issued, a powerful magnifying glass included in every slipcase. Then came a CD-ROM, and not long afterward the great work was further adapted for use on-line. A third edition, with a vast budget, was in the works.

There is some occasional carping that the work reflects an elitist, male, British, Victorian tone. Yet even in the admission that, like so many achievements of the era, it did reflect a set of attitudes not wholly harmonic with those prevalent at the end of the twentieth century, none seem to suggest that any other dictionary has ever come close, or will ever come close, to the achievement that it offers. It was the heroic creation of a legion of interested and enthusiastic men and women of wide general knowledge and interest; and it lives on today, just as lives the language of which it rightly claims to be a portrait.

Postscript

Memorial (mǐmōᵊ·riăl), *a.* and *sb.* [a. OF. *memo-rial* (mod.F. *mémorial*) = Sp., Pg. *memorial*, It. *me-moriale*, ad. L. *memoriālis* adj. (neut. *memoriāle*, used in late Latin as sb.), f. *memoria* MEMORY.]
A. adj.
  1. Preserving the memory of a person or thing;
  3. Something by which the memory of a person, thing, or event is preserved, as a monumental erection

This has been the story of an American soldier whose involvement in the making of the world's greatest dictionary was singular, astonishing, memorable, and laudable—and yet at the same time wretchedly sad. And in the telling, it is tempting to forget that the circumstances that placed William Chester Minor in the position in which he was able to contribute all his time and energy to the making of the *OED* began with his horrible and unforgivable commission of a murder.

George Merrett, who was his victim, was an ordinary, innocent working-class farmer's son from Wiltshire, who came up to London to make his living but who was shot dead, leaving a pregnant wife, Eliza, and seven young children. The family was already living in the direst poverty, trying to maintain some semblance of their farm-country dignity amid the squalor of one of the roughest and most unforgiving parts of the Victorian city. With Merrett's murder matters took a terrible turn for the worse.

All London was shocked and horrified by the killing, and funds were raised and money collected to help the widow and her brood. Americans in particular, stunned by the outrage committed by one of their own, were asked by their consul-general to contribute to a diplomatic fund; the vicars in Lambeth banded together to make collections, ecumenically; a series of amateur entertainments—including one "of an unusually high-class character" with readings of Longfellow and of a selection from *Othello*, and held at the Hercules Club—were staged across town to raise money; and the funeral itself was a splendid affair, as impressive as that of any grandee.

George Merrett had been a member of the Ancient Order of Foresters—one of the many so-called friendly societies that were once popular across Britain—as a means, in the absence of any government or privately funded schemes, of providing cooperative pensions and other financial help for the working classes. On the night he died Merrett had been relieving a shift worker who was a brother Forester: This small act of benevolence doubly obliged the order to offer its late member a handsome farewell.

The cortége was half a mile long: The Foresters' band playing the Dead March from *Saul* came first, then scores of emblem-wearing members, then the horse-drawn hearse and four black mourning coaches to carry the bereaved. Eliza Merrett rode in the lead carriage, holding her youngest baby in her arms and sobbing. Hundreds of brewery workers followed, and then thousands of ordinary members of the public, all wearing black crepe bands around their arms or hats.

For the entire afternoon the procession wound from Lambeth, past the spot on Belvedere Road where the tragedy had occurred, past the Bedlam Hospital, and up to the vast cemetery at Tooting, where George Merrett was finally buried.

His grave may once have been marked, but it lacks a marker now, and where the records say George Merrett lies there is no more than a patch of discolored grass, a tiny patch of settled earth among a sea of more nobler and newer monuments.

As we have seen, in his lucid moments William Minor was contrite, appalled by the consequences of his moment of mad delusion. From his cells at Broadmoor he saw to it that money was sent to the family to help them in their distress. His stepmother, Judith, had already arranged gifts for the children. Some seven years after the tragedy, when Minor wrote to express his remorse, Eliza Merrett said that she forgave him, and she made what now seems the extraordinary decision to visit him in Broadmoor—and indeed for some months came down to Crowthorne frequently and brought him packages of his beloved books. But she never really recovered from the shock of what had happened: Before long she had taken to drink, and when she died it was of liver failure.

Two of her sons' lives then unraveled most curiously: George, the second oldest boy, took Judith's gift of money to Monaco, won a considerable sum, and remained there, styling himself the king of Monte Carlo, before dying in impoverished obscurity in the south of France. His younger brother Frederick shot himself dead in London, for reasons that have never been fully explained. The fact that two of Minor's brothers also died by their own hand invests the entire story with almost more sadness than is bearable.

But the principal tragic figure in this strange tale is the man who is the least well remembered—the one who was gunned down on the damp and cold cobblestones of Lambeth on that Saturday night in February 1872.

The only public memorials ever raised to the two most tragically linked of this saga's protagonists are miserable, niggardly affairs. William Minor has just a simple little gravestone in a New Haven cemetery, hemmed in between litter and slums. George Merrett has for years had nothing at all, except for a patch of grayish grass in a sprawling graveyard in South London. Minor does, however, have the advantage of the great dictionary, which some might say acts as his most lasting remembrance. But nothing else remains to suggest that the man he killed was ever worthy of any memory at all. George Merrett has become an absolutely unsung man.

Which is why it now seems fitting, more than a century and a quarter on, that this modest account begins with the dedication that it does. And why this book is offered as a small testament to the late George Merrett of Wiltshire and Lambeth, without whose untimely death these events would never have unfolded, and this tale could never have been told.

Author's Note

|| **Coda** (kō·da, kōu·dă). *Mus.* [Ital.:–L. *cauda* tail.] A passage of more or less independent character introduced after the completion of the essential parts of a movement, so as to form a more definite and satisfactory conclusion.

I first became intrigued by the central figure of this story, the dictionary itself, back in the early 1980s, when I was living in Oxford. One summer's day a friend who worked at the university press invited me into a warehouse to look at a forgotten treasure. It was a jumbled pile of metal plates, each one measuring a little more than seven inches by ten, and—as I found when I picked one up—as heavy as the devil.

They were the discarded letterpress printing plates from which the *Oxford English Dictionary* had been made. The original lead-fronted, steel-and-antimony-backed plates, cast in the nineteenth and early twentieth centuries, from which all the many printings of the *OED*—from the individual fascicles made as the books were being edited, to the final twelve-volume masterpiece of 1928—had been made.

The press, my friend explained, had recently adopted more modern methods: computer typesetting, photolithography, and the like. The old ways of the letterpress men—with their slugs of lead and their typesticks, their em-quads and their brasses and coppers, their tympan paper and their platen brushes and their uncanny ability to read backward and upside down at speed—were at long last being abandoned. The plates, and all the job-cases of type for hand-setting, were now being tossed away, melted down, carried off.

Would I perhaps like one or two of the plates, he asked me—just to keep as souvenirs of something that had once been rather marvelous?

I chose three of them, reading the backward type as best I could in the dim and dusty light. Two of them I later gave away. But I kept one: It was the complete page 452 of the great dictionary's volume 5: It encompassed the words *humoral* to *humour*, it had been edited in 1901 or so, and set in type in 1902.

For years I took the strange, dirty-looking old plate around with me. It was a kind of talisman. I would squirrel it away in cupboards in the various flats and houses in the various cities and villages in which I came to live. I was rather proud of it—boringly so, I dare say—and every so often I would find it hidden behind other, more important things, and I would bring it out, blow off the dust, and show it off to friends, a small and fascinating item of lexicographic history.

I am sure at first they thought I was a little mad—though in truth I fancy they seemed after a while to understand my odd affection for the blackened—and *so heavy!*—little thing. I would watch as they rubbed their fingers gently over its raised lead, and nod in mute agreement: The plate seemed to offer them some kind of tactile pleasure, as well as a simpler intellectual amusement.

When I came to live in the United States in the mid-nineties, I met a letterpress printer, a woman who lived in western Massachusetts. I told her about the plate, and she became visibly excited. She had a great enthusiasm for the story of the making of the dictionary, she said, as well as a tremendous fondness for its design—for the elegant and clever mix of typography and font sizes the stern old Victorian editors had employed. She asked to see my plate, and when I brought it to her, she asked if she might borrow it for a while.

That while turned into two long years, during which time she took on as much other work as a hand printer gets these days. She embarked on a series of broadsides for John Updike, made chapbooks for a couple of other New England poets, published a collection or two of short stories and plays, all of which she had printed on handmade paper. She was very much the craftswoman, all her work meticulous, slow, perfect. And she kept my dictionary plate standing on a windowsill all the while, wondering what best to do with it.

Finally she decided. She knew that I had a great liking for China and had lived there for many years; and that I was also fonder of Oxford than any other English city. So she took down the plate; washed it carefully in a range of solvents to purge it of its accumulated dust, grease, and ink; mounted it on her Vandercook proof printer; and carefully pressed, on the finest handwoven paper, two editions of the page—one inked in Oxford blue, the other in China red.

She then mounted the three items side by side—the metal plate in the middle, the red page to the left, the other, blue page to the right—and set them inside a slender gold frame behind nonreflecting glass. She left the completed picture, with wire and bracket for hanging it on the wall, in a small café in her hometown, and then wrote a postcard telling me to pick it up whenever I could, and at the same time to take care to enjoy the café owner's strawberry-rhubarb pie and her cappuccino. There was no bill, and I have never seen the printer since.

But the plate and its proof sheets hang on my wall still, above a small lamp that illuminates an open volume of the great dictionary on the desk below. It is volume 5, and I keep it open to the same page that was once printed from the actual piece of metal that hangs suspended just above it. It is what Victorians would have called a grand conjunction, and it serves as a small shrine to the pleasures of bookmaking and printing, and to the joy of words.

Once my mother noticed that the dominant entry on the plate and the sheets and in the book below is the word *humorist*. It reminded her of a nicely droll coincidence, another conjunction, though one rather less grand. *Humorist* had been the name of a horse that ran in the Derby on June 1, 1921, the day my mother was born. Her father, so pleased at the news of the birth of a baby girl, had put ten guineas on the filly, rank outsider though she was. But she won, and a grandfather I never met made a thousand guineas, all because of a word that briefly took his fancy.

Acknowledgments

Acknowledgment (ăknǫ·lėdʒmĕnt); also **acknowledgement** (a spelling more in accordance with Eng. values of letters). [f. ACKNOWLEDGE *v.* + -MENT. An early instance of *-ment* added to an orig. Eng. vb.]

1. The act of acknowledging, confessing, admitting, or owning; confession, avowal.

5. The owning of a gift or benefit received, or of a message; grateful, courteous, or due recognition.

6. Hence, The sensible sign, whereby anything received is acknowledged; something given or done in return for a favour or message, or a formal communication that we have received it.

1739 T. SHERIDAN *Persius* Ded. 3, I dedicate to you this Edition and Translation of Persius, as an Acknowledgment for the great Pleasure you gave me. **1802** MAR. EDGEWORTH *Moral T.* (1816) I. xvi. 133 To offer him some acknowledgment for his obliging conduct. **1881** *Daily Tel.* Dec. 27 The painter had to appear and bow his acknowledgments. *Mod.* Take this as a small acknowledgement of my gratitude.

When I first came upon this story, which was mentioned all too briefly, and just as an aside, in a rather sober book about the dictionary-making craft, it struck me immediately as a tale well worth investigating and perhaps telling in full. But for several months I was alone in thinking so. I had in the works a truly massive project about an altogether different subject, and the advice from virtually all sides was that I should press on with that and leave this amusing little saga well alone.

But four people did find it just as fascinating as I did—and saw also the possibilities that by telling the poignant and human tale of William Minor, I could perhaps create some kind of prism through which to view the greater and even more fascinating story of the history of English lexicography. These four people were Bill Hamilton, my longtime friend and London agent; Anya Waddington, my editor at Viking, also in London; Larry Ashmead, Executive Editor of Harper-Collins in New York; and Marisa Milanese, then an editorial assistant in the offices of *Condé Nast Traveler* magazine, also in New York. Their faith in this otherwise unregarded project was total and unremitting, and I thank them for it unreservedly.

Marisa, whom I think a paragon of ceaseless enthusiasm, dogged initiative, and untiring zeal, then went on to help me with the American end of the research: Together with my close friend of a quarter century, Juliet Walker in London, she helped me spin my basic ideas into a complex web of facts and figures, which I have since attempted to settle into some kind of coherent order. The extent to which I have succeeded or failed in this I cannot yet judge, but I should say here that these two women presented me with a bottomless well of information, and if I have misinterpreted, misread, misheard, or miswritten any of it, then those mistakes are my responsibility, and mine alone. My thanks also to Sue Llewellyn, who, as well as copyediting this book so assiduously and with such good humor, also—she reminded me—had worked on my book on Korea ten years before.

Access to Broadmoor Special Hospital, and to the voluminous files that have long been kept on all patients, was clearly going to be the key to cracking this story; and it took some weeks before Juliet Walker and I were allowed in. That we were was a triumph for two Broadmoor employees, Paul Robertson and Alison Webster, who made a persuasive case on our behalf to a perhaps understandably reluctant hospital administration. Without the help of these two remarkable and kind individuals, this book would never have managed to be much more than a collection of conjectures: The Broadmoor files were needed to provide the facts, and Paul and Alison provided the files.

On the other side of the Atlantic, matters proceeded rather differently—despite the best efforts of the splendid Marisa. St. Elizabeth's Hospital in Washington, D.C., is no longer a federal institution but is run by the government of the District of Columbia—a government that has experienced some well-publicized troubles in recent years. And at first, perhaps because of this, the hospital refused point-blank to release any of its files, and went so far as to suggest, quite seriously, that I engage a lawyer and sue in order to obtain them.

However, some while later, a cursory search I made one day of the National Archives pages on the World Wide Web suggested to me that the papers relating to Doctor Minor— who had been a patient at St. Elizabeth's between 1910 and 1919, when the institution was undeniably under federal jurisdiction—might well actually be in federal custody, and not within the Kafkaesque embrace of the District. And indeed, as it turned out, they were. A couple of requests through the Internet, a happy conversation with the extremely helpful archivist Bill Breach, and suddenly more than seven hundred pages of case notes and other fascinating miscellanea arrived in a FedEx package. It was more than gratifying to be able to telephone St. Elizabeth's the next day and tell the unhelpful officials there which file I then had sitting before me on my desk. They were not best pleased.

The Oxford University Press was, by contrast, wonderfully helpful; and while I am naturally happy to thank the officials at the press who so kindly sanctioned my visits to Walton Street, I wish to acknowledge the very considerable debt that I owe first to Elizabeth Knowles, now of Oxford's Reference Books Department, who had made a study of Minor some years before and was happy to share her knowledge and access with me. I am delighted also to be able to thank the irrepressibly enthusiastic Jenny McMorris of the press archives, who knows Minor and his remarkable legacy more intimately than anyone else anywhere. Jenny, together with her former colleague Peter Foden, proved a tower of strength during my visits and long after: I only hope that she manages to find an outlet for her own fascination with the great Dr. Henry Fowler, whom she rightly regards, along with Murray, as one of the true heroes of the English language.

Several friends, as well as a number of specialists who had a professional interest in parts of the story, were kind enough to read the manuscript's early drafts, and they made many suggestions for improving it. In almost all cases I have accepted their proposals with gratitude, but if on occasion I did, through carelessness or pigheadedness, disregard their warnings or demands, then the same caveat—about the responsibility for all errors of fact, judgment, or taste remaining firmly with me—applies as well: They did their best.

Among those personal friends I wish to thank are Graham Boynton, Pepper Evans, Rob Howard, Jesse Sheidlower, Nancy Stump, Paula Szuchman, and Gully Wells. And to the otherwise anonymous Anthony S——, who grumbled to me that his fiancée had denied him romantic favors one summer morning because she was bent on finishing chapter 9, my apologies, embarrassed thanks for your forbearance, and best wishes for future marital bliss.

James W. Campbell of the New Haven Historical Society gave great assistance in finding the Minor family in their old hometown; the librarians and staff at the Yale Divinity Library told me much about William Minor's early life in Ceylon. Pat Higgins, an Englishwoman living in Washington State, and with whom I corresponded only by e-mail, became fascinated also by the Ceylon and Seattle ends of the Minor family story and gave me several fascinating tips.

Michael Musick of the U.S. National Archives then found most of Minor's military files, and Michael Rhode of the Walter Reed Army Hospital tracked down his handwritten autopsy reports. The National Park Service was helpful in giving me access to military bases in New York and Florida where he had been stationed; the Index Project in Arlington, Va., assisted me in finding additional records relating to his wartime career.

Susan Pakies of Virginia's Orange County Tourist Office, along with the immensely knowledgeable Frank Walker, then took me around all of the important sites where the Battle of the Wilderness had been fought, and later, to cheer us all up, to several of the delightful old inns that are hidden away in this spectacularly lovely corner of the United States. Jonathan O'Neal patiently explained Civil War medical practice at the old Exchange Hotel-cum-hospital that is now a museum in Gordonville, Va.

Nancy Whitmore of the National Museum of Civil War Medicine in Frederick, Maryland, was an enthusiastic supporter of the project and painstakingly dug up a huge amount of highly relevant arcana. Dr. Lawrence Kohl at the University of Alabama was kind enough to take time both to discuss the mechanics of Civil War branding and to speculate (in an impressively informed way) on the effects such punishment might have had on Irishmen who fought in the Union Army—the latter his particular specialty as a historian of the period. Mitchell Redman of New York City filled in some details of Minor's later personal life, about which he had once written a short but so far unproduced play.

Gordon Claridge of Magdalen College, Oxford, had much that was helpful to say about the origins of mental illness; Jonathan Andrews, a historian of Broadmoor, helped also; and Isa Samad, a distinguished psychiatrist of Fort Lauderdale, Fla., told me a great deal about the history of the treatment of paranoid schizophrenia.

Dale Fiore, superintendent of the Evergreen Cemetery in New Haven, then added fascinating footnotes about the end of William Minor's life—the length of the coffin, the depth at which it is buried, and the names of those who surround him in his plot.

Life became a great deal easier once I had tracked down one of the few known living relatives of William Minor, Mr. John Minor, of Riverside, Conn. He was kindness itself, giving me an enormous amount of useful information about the great-great-uncle he never knew, and offering me access to the treasure trove of pictures and papers that had sat for years, undisturbed, in a wooden box in his attic. He and his Danish wife, Birgit, became as fascinated by the story as I was, and I thank them for pleasant waterside dinners and time spent talking about the nature of their most curious relative.

David Merritt of the Merritt International Family History Society [sic] in London gave me valuable help in ferreting out details of where George Merrett's descendants might be: I eventually found one, a Mr. Dean Blanchard in Sussex, who was equally interested in the fortunes of his distant family, and shared much that was valuable with me.

I am indebted also to my American agent, Peter Matson; his colleague Jennifer Hengen; and to Agnes Krup, who, once enthused by the strange nature of this story, became among its keenest supporters and kept me going, writing hard, during a long hot American summer. My wife, Catherine, saw to it that I remained undisturbed, and offered generously the kind of serenity and sanctuary that the writing of a yarn like this more than amply deserves.

Suggestions for Further Reading

The book that first inspired me to look into this story was Jonathon Green's *Chasing the Sun* (Jonathan Cape, London, and Henry Holt, New York, 1996), which devoted a page and a half to the tale, and led me, via its bibliography, to the rather more celebrated work about the making of the *OED*, *Caught in the Web of Words* (Oxford and Yale University Presses, 1977), written by the great editor's granddaughter, K. M. Elisabeth Murray. In both cases the tale of the first meeting between Murray and Minor relies on the well-known myth; but it was not until Elizabeth Knowles wrote a more accurate account in the quarterly journal *Dictionaries* that some of the truth of the encounter became more properly known. Both of the books will delight the enthusiast; the journal tends toward the academic, but since—at least superficially—the disciplines of lexicography are frankly not too taxing, many may profit from looking at it as well.

For those interested in the basic principles behind the making of word books, Sidney Landau's definitive *Dictionaries— The Art and Craft of Lexicography* (Charles Scribner's Sons, New York, 1984) is an essential read. For those iconoclasts wishing to understand the flaws in the *OED*, John Willinsky explains much in his rather ill-tempered *Empire of Words— The Reign of the OED* (Princeton University Press, 1994), which offers a politically correct revisionist view of James Murray's creation—albeit from a somewhat admiring stance. It is worth reading, even if just to make one's blood boil.

Copies of Doctor Johnson's *Dictionary* can usually still be found quite easily—reproductions of the large-format two-volume editions have been produced on presses in such unlikely settings as the city of Beirut, from where I recently purchased a copy for $250. It is difficult to find a good first edition for under $15,000. But there is a witty and useful distillation, with words selected by E. L. McAdam and George Milne (Pantheon, New York, 1963; paperback reprint, Cassell, London, 1995).

The Oxford University Press deserves a history of its own, and indeed has several: I recommend Peter Sutcliffe's *The Oxford University Press: An Informal History* (Oxford University Press, 1978), which covers the saga of the making of the *OED* very well, and with reasonable impartiality.

The American Civil War is of course very comprehensively covered. The best book relating to the fighting in which Doctor Minor played a small but, for him, crucial part, is Gordon C. Rhea's *The Battle of the Wilderness* (Louisiana State University Press, 1994), which I enjoyed enormously. D. P. Conyngham's 1867 classic *The Irish Brigade and its Campaigns* has recently been reissued (Fordham University Press, New York, 1994), with an introduction by Lawrence F. Kohl, whose help with my own book I acknowledge elsewhere. Among the many books on Civil War medicine I enjoyed George Worthington Adams's *Doctors in Blue* (Louisiana State University Press, 1980) and *In Hospital and Camp* by

Harold Elk Straubing (Stackpole Books, Harrisburg, Pa., 1993). I also took time to read the relevant chapters in that elegant giant of a book *The American Heritage New History of the Civil War,* by Bruce Catton and James M. Macpherson (Viking, New York, 1996), which answers practically every imaginable question about the minutiae of those four years of bloody fighting.

The nature of the possible mental ailments that plagued Doctor Minor, which may have been triggered by his experiences during the war, are comprehensively explained by Gordon Claridge in *Origins of Mental Illness* (ISHK Malor Books, Cambridge, Mass., 1995). Andrew Scull's splendid *Masters of Bedlam* (Princeton University Press, 1996) offers a fascinating history of the mad-doctoring trade before the times of psychiatric enlightenment.

I looked to Roy Porter—also an expert on madness and its treatment—for his rightly acclaimed social history of the city where Minor committed his murder: *London: A Social History* (Harvard, 1994) sets the scene admirably, and remains one of the best books on England's remarkable capital.

But the one book that above all should be read in conjunction with this small volume is one of the biggest and most impressive works of scholarship to be found—the twelve-volume first edition, the 1933 supplement, the four supplementary volumes of Robert Burchfield, or the fully integrated twenty-volume *Second Edition of The Oxford English Dictionary* itself.

It makes for an expensive and bulky set of books—which is why nowadays the CD-ROM is much preferred—but it

does, most important of all to his fans, acknowledge formally the existence and contributions of Doctor Minor. And
I find that somehow the simple discovery of his name, buried as it is among those of the contributors who helped make
the *OED* the great totem that it remains today, is always an
intensely touching moment.

While it is of course in and of itself no justification for
ever needing to own the great book, the finding of Minor's
name presents perhaps the finest of examples of the kind of
serendipitous moment for which the *OED* is justly famous.
And few would disagree that serendipity, in dictionaries, is a
most splendid thing indeed.

COOL PAPERBACKS, COOL PRICE

How to Be a Woman	*You Learn by Living*	*Profiles in Courage*	*The Orchardist*
Caitlin Moran	Eleanor Roosevelt	John F. Kennedy	Amanda Coplin

OLIVE EDITIONS for $10 EACH

Available for a Limited Time Only

The Space Between Us	*So Big*	*Pilgrim at Tinker Creek*	*The Professor and the Madman*
Thrity Umrigar	Edna Ferber	Annie Dillard	Simon Winchester

Available for a limited time wherever books are sold, or call 1-800-331-3761 to order.